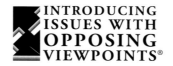

INTRODUCING ISSUES WITH OPPOSING VIEWPOINTS®

AIDS

Mary E. Williams, *Book Editor*

GREENHAVEN PRESS

A part of Gale, Cengage Learning

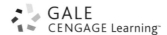

GALE
CENGAGE Learning™

Detroit • New York • San Francisco • New Haven, Conn • Waterville, Maine • London

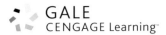

Christine Nasso, *Publisher*
Elizabeth Des Chenes, *Managing Editor*

© 2011 Greenhaven Press, a part of Gale, Cengage Learning

Gale and Greenhaven Press are registered trademarks used herein under license.

For more information, contact:
Greenhaven Press
27500 Drake Rd.
Farmington Hills, MI 48331-3535
Or you can visit our Internet site at gale.cengage.com

For product information and technology assistance, contact us at

Gale Customer Support, 1-800-877-4253
For permission to use material from this text or product, submit all requests online at www.cengage.com/permissions

Further permissions questions can be e-mailed to permissionrequest@cengage.com

Articles in Greenhaven Press anthologies are often edited for length to meet page requirements. In addition, original titles of these works are changed to clearly present the main thesis and to explicitly indicate the author's opinion. Every effort is made to ensure that Greenhaven Press accurately reflects the original intent of the authors. Every effort has been made to trace the owners of copyrighted material.

Cover image copyright © Travelshots/Travelshots.com/Alamy.

LIBRARY OF CONGRESS CATALOGING-IN-PUBLICATION DATA

AIDS / Mary E. Williams, book editor.
    p. cm. -- (Introducing issues with opposing viewpoints)
  Includes bibliographical references and index.
  ISBN 978-0-7377-5197-0 (hardcover)
  1. AIDS (Disease)--Epidemiology. 2. AIDS (Disease)--Prevention. 3. AIDS (Disease)--Government policy. I. Williams, Mary E., 1960-
  RA643.8.A32 2011
  614.5'99392--dc22

                  2010045538

Printed in the United States of America
1 2 3 4 5 6 7 15 14 13 12 11

Contents

Foreword

Indulging in a wide spectrum of ideas, beliefs, and perspectives is a critical cornerstone of democracy. After all, it is often debates over differences of opinion, such as whether to legalize abortion, how to treat prisoners, or when to enact the death penalty, that shape our society and drive it forward. Such diversity of thought is frequently regarded as the hallmark of a healthy and civilized culture. As the Reverend Clifford Schutjer of the First Congregational Church in Mansfield, Ohio, declared in a 2001 sermon, "Surrounding oneself with only like-minded people, restricting what we listen to or read only to what we find agreeable is irresponsible. Refusing to entertain doubts once we make up our minds is a subtle but deadly form of arrogance." With this advice in mind, Introducing Issues with Opposing Viewpoints books aim to open readers' minds to the critically divergent views that comprise our world's most important debates.

Introducing Issues with Opposing Viewpoints simplifies for students the enormous and often overwhelming mass of material now available via print and electronic media. Collected in every volume is an array of opinions that captures the essence of a particular controversy or topic. Introducing Issues with Opposing Viewpoints books embody the spirit of nineteenth-century journalist Charles A. Dana's axiom: "Fight for your opinions, but do not believe that they contain the whole truth, or the only truth." Absorbing such contrasting opinions teaches students to analyze the strength of an argument and compare it to its opposition. From this process readers can inform and strengthen their own opinions, or be exposed to new information that will change their minds. Introducing Issues with Opposing Viewpoints is a mosaic of different voices. The authors are statesmen, pundits, academics, journalists, corporations, and ordinary people who have felt compelled to share their experiences and ideas in a public forum. Their words have been collected from newspapers, journals, books, speeches, interviews, and the Internet, the fastest growing body of opinionated material in the world.

Introducing Issues with Opposing Viewpoints shares many of the well-known features of its critically acclaimed parent series, Opposing Viewpoints. The articles are presented in a pro/con format, allowing readers to absorb divergent perspectives side by side. Active reading questions preface each viewpoint, requiring the student to approach the material thoughtfully and carefully. Useful charts, graphs, and cartoons supplement each article. A thorough introduction provides readers with crucial background on an issue. An annotated bibliography points the reader toward articles, books, and websites that contain additional information on the topic. An appendix of organizations to contact contains a wide variety of charities, nonprofit organizations, political groups, and private enterprises that each hold a position on the issue at hand. Finally, a comprehensive index allows readers to locate content quickly and efficiently.

Introducing Issues with Opposing Viewpoints is also significantly different from Opposing Viewpoints. As the series title implies, its presentation will help introduce students to the concept of opposing viewpoints and learn to use this material to aid in critical writing and debate. The series' four-color, accessible format makes the books attractive and inviting to readers of all levels. In addition, each viewpoint has been carefully edited to maximize a reader's understanding of the content. Short but thorough viewpoints capture the essence of an argument. A substantial, thought-provoking essay question placed at the end of each viewpoint asks the student to further investigate the issues raised in the viewpoint, compare and contrast two authors' arguments, or consider how one might go about forming an opinion on the topic at hand. Each viewpoint contains sidebars that include at-a-glance information and handy statistics. A Facts About section located in the back of the book further supplies students with relevant facts and figures.

Following in the tradition of the Opposing Viewpoints series, Greenhaven Press continues to provide readers with invaluable exposure to the controversial issues that shape our world. As John Stuart Mill once wrote: "The only way in which a human being can make some approach to knowing the whole of a subject is by hearing what can be said about it by persons of every variety of opinion and studying all modes in which it can be looked at by every character of mind. No wise man ever acquired his wisdom in any mode but this." It is to this principle that Introducing Issues with Opposing Viewpoints books are dedicated.

Introduction

"Challenges to successful [HIV] treatment include getting people tested, getting people to adhere to treatment, having the necessary infrastructure and workforce to deliver treatment, and reaching patients regardless of location or other barrier."

—Matthew Leake, Avert.org, June 2009.

It was June 1981 when the Centers for Disease Control first announced the discovery of a dangerous new disease, AIDS (an acronym for acquired immunodeficiency syndrome). AIDS is caused by infection with HIV (the human immunodeficiency virus), a retrovirus that attacks the immune system and eventually results in death through illnesses normally repelled by the body's natural defenses. Initially determining that the disease is transmitted sexually, researchers later learned that AIDS is also spread through contaminated blood and from mother to child during pregnancy and breast-feeding.

There was a high level of alarm and confusion during the first years of the AIDS epidemic. In the United States HIV was first identified in gay men. Because of the initial uncertainty about how AIDS actually spread, people infected with HIV faced stigma and discrimination in schools, in workplaces, in hospitals, and at national borders. Between 1983 and 1986 major outbreaks of AIDS were reported in central Africa, India, and Russia, and the global health community recognized that a pandemic was in the making. In 1986 the US surgeon general mailed information on AIDS to every household in an effort to educate the American public on preventative measures. The following year the first anti-AIDS drug, AZT, was developed.

Just one decade after the discovery of AIDS, in 1991 the World Health Organization (WHO) estimated that 10 million people had become infected with HIV. By the year 2001 more than 20 million people worldwide had died of complications resulting from AIDS, and the disease had become the leading cause of death in sub-Saharan Africa. Despite these devastating statistics, however, there were some hopeful signs in the arena of AIDS research, prevention, and treatment. Quicker, more accurate HIV tests had been developed. A variety of pharmaceutical "cocktails"—antiretroviral therapies that combine three or more drugs—were enabling HIV-positive people to live longer and healthier lives than those who had succumbed in the early years of the epidemic. In addition, educational and preventative campaigns were proving successful in some countries. After the beginning of the new millennium, many Western nations were actually seeing a decline in their numbers of new AIDS cases. This decline was likely the result of enhanced awareness about HIV testing and prevention as well as access to drug therapies that increase the number of years before HIV infection progresses into full-blown AIDS.

The situation in much of the world remains stark, however. In 2009 more than 33 million people worldwide were living with HIV/AIDS—the great majority of them residents of middle- and low-income countries. According to a joint study conducted by the WHO, the Joint United Nations Programme on HIV/AIDS, and the United Nations Children's Fund, 5.25 million people in poorer nations had access to HIV treatment in 2009, accounting for 36 percent of those in need of it. Funding shortages, limited human resources, and poorly organized health-care systems have kept needed diagnostics and drugs from reaching some of the more hard-hit regions of the world. The global health community continues to push for universal access to HIV prevention, treatment, and care. "The number of people receiving HIV antiretroviral therapy (ART) in low- and middle-income countries increased from 400,000 in 2003 to 4 million in 2008," writes Robin Gorna, executive director of the International AIDS Society in the spring 2010 *Global Health* magazine. "That's good progress, but we're still only reaching about one-third of the people who need HIV therapy today. . . . Of course, on an individual level, every person reached with ART or with the tools and information to avoid HIV infection is a victory. Globally, however, the only way to reduce and ultimately end this epidemic is to reach a very high level of people in need."

Epidemiologist and researcher Brian Williams argues that even more needs to be done. Currently, he points out, antiretroviral drugs are administered to people too late in the course of their HIV infection. This may prolong their lives, but it does not reduce HIV transmission rates. Williams maintains that very early detection and treatment could actually stop the spread of HIV: "[There are] extremely effective drugs that keep people alive and reduce their viral load by up to 2000 times. They become close to non-infectious." Early treatment of HIV might become as effective as a vaccine would be in preventing the spread of AIDS. "We could break the back of the epidemic," said Williams in a February 2010 BBC interview.

Not everyone agrees that universal access to HIV testing and treatment is the best way to slow the spread of AIDS. For one thing, universal access does not lead to universal compliance. For a variety of reasons, some of those who receive antiretroviral drugs discontinue treatment or do not take the drugs consistently. This could lead to the development of drug-resistant strains of HIV. Moreover, some experts argue, easy access to anti-AIDS drugs could create a sense of complacency about the disease. "The problem with HIV is that it is both an infectious disease and a behavioral one," notes researcher Elizabeth Pisani in the September 25, 2009, edition of *The Times* (London). "Will [pills or a vaccine] make me more likely to share needles, or less likely to use condoms?" She notes that after HIV treatment became universally available in England, "condom use in the gay community fell and new HIV infections rose, even though treatment greatly reduces the risk of passing the virus on." For these reasons, some experts believe that educational efforts focusing on prevention and individual responsibility are preferable to universal access programs.

How to best curtail the global AIDS pandemic is perhaps the most challenging question surrounding AIDS and international health policy today. Through their debates about the significance of HIV as a public health threat and their various approaches to controlling its transmission, the authors in *Introducing Issues with Opposing Viewpoints: AIDS* provide a thought-provoking overview of this evolving controversy.

Chapter 1

How Serious a Threat Is the AIDS Epidemic?

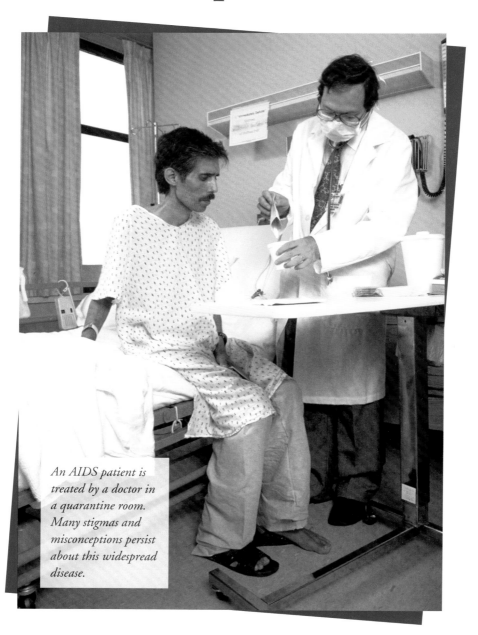

An AIDS patient is treated by a doctor in a quarantine room. Many stigmas and misconceptions persist about this widespread disease.

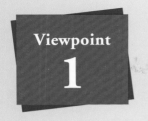

The Number of AIDS Deaths Is Decreasing

Global Agenda

"As treatment programmes are installed around the world, death rates are falling."

In the following selection the editors of the yearly journal *Global Agenda* maintain that the worldwide AIDS epidemic is not as bad as it once seemed. Although the epidemic remains devastating and the number of HIV infections has risen, AIDS death rates have actually fallen. New counting methods show that fewer people have AIDS than previously thought, the authors report. In addition, education and improved medical treatment are enabling those infected with HIV to survive longer than they did in the past.

AS YOU READ, CONSIDER THE FOLLOWING QUESTIONS:
1. In what year did the death rate from AIDS peak, according to *Global Agenda*?
2. According to the authors, what was the highest annual number of new HIV infections? In what year did this occur?
3. Which improvements in survey methods resulted in more accurate data about the AIDS epidemic, according to this viewpoint?

On the face of things, a fall in the number of people infected with HIV (the virus that causes AIDS) from 39.5 [million] to 33.2 [million] over the course of a single year should be cause for rejoicing. That is the news from this year's AIDS epidemic update from the World Health Organisation (WHO) and UNAIDS [Joint United Nations Programme on HIV/AIDS] published on Tuesday November 20th [2007]. Indeed, it is good news, for it means there are fewer people to treat, and fewer to pass the infection on, than was previously thought. But the fall is not a real fall. Rather, it is due to a change in the way the size of the epidemic is estimated.

Factor that change in and the number of infected individuals has actually risen since last year [2006], by 500,000. And even that is not necessarily bad news in the paradoxical world of AIDS. As treatment programmes are installed around the world, death rates are falling. According to the revised figures, the peak, of 2.2 [million] a year, was in 2005. Now the figure is 2.1 [million]. Since the only way for an infected person to drop out of the statistics in reality (as opposed to by sleight of statistical hand) is for him to die, such increased survivorship inevitably pushes up the total size of the epidemic.

The Epidemic Has Peaked

The best news of all, however, is that the new figures confirm what had previously been suspected—that the epidemic has peaked. The highest annual number of new infections around the world was 3.4 [million] in 1998. That figure has now fallen to 2.5 [million].

Both the change in the death rate and the change in the infection rate are partly a consequence of the natural flow and ebb of any epidemic infection. But the changes are also a reflection of the hard graft of public-health workers in many countries, which has persuaded people to modify or abandon risky behaviour, such as having unpro-

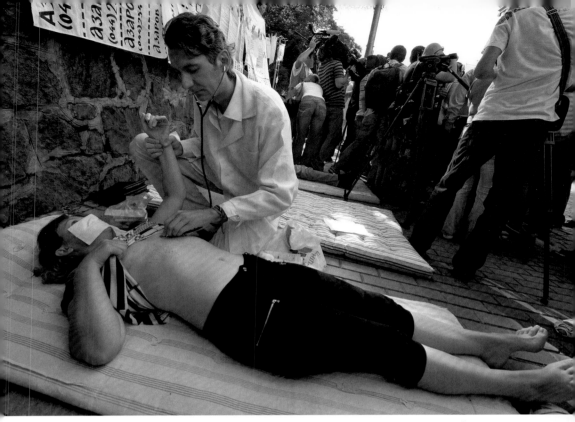

A doctor treats an AIDS patient in Ukraine in 2010. As treatment programs become available around the world, death rates are falling.

tected sex, and has also created the medical infrastructure needed to distribute anti-retroviral drugs that can keep symptoms at bay in those who do become infected.

The revision of the figures is mainly a result of better data-collection methods, particularly in India (which accounts for half the downward revision) and five African countries (which account for another fifth). In India many more sampling points have been established, and in all countries better survey methods, relying on surveyors knocking on doors rather than asking questions at clinics, have gathered data from more representative samples of the population.

The Need for Accurate Data

Sceptics will feel vindicated by the revision. There has been a feeling around for a while that the older survey methods were biased, and that the inflation thus produced was tolerated because it helped twang the heart-strings of potential donors. However, the structures

HIV in Sub-Saharan Africa

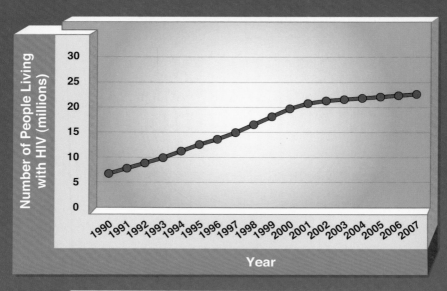

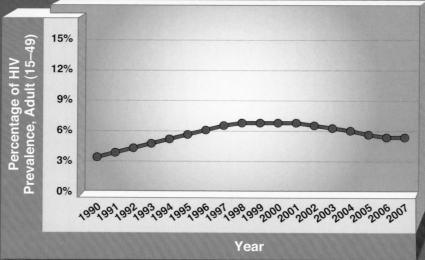

Note: Even though the HIV prevalence stabilized in sub-Saharan Africa, the actual number of people infected continues to grow because of new infections.

Taken from: Taken from: UNAIDS, *HIV Global Report,* 2008. www.unaids.org/en/knowledgecentre/HIVData/Global Report/2008/2008/Global.report.asp.

for collecting and distributing money to combat AIDS are now well established, and accurate data are crucial if that money is not to be misdirected.

The new information also means that the goal of treatment for all who need it will be easier and cheaper to achieve. The WHO and UNAIDS are planning to publish a report on the matter early next year [2008] but Paul De Lay, UNAIDS's director of evidence, monitoring and policy, says that the financial requirements for 2010 will probably be about 5% less than previously estimated, and by 2015 that figure will have risen to 10%. Good news for everyone, then, donors and sufferers alike.

EVALUATING THE AUTHOR'S ARGUMENTS:

As *Global Agenda* points out, statistics about AIDS can be misleading. Why is the fall in the number of people infected with HIV not a "real fall"? How is it that a decrease in the number of AIDS deaths statistically increases the total size of the epidemic? Do you agree with the author that new estimates about the global AIDS epidemic is "good news"? Why or why not?

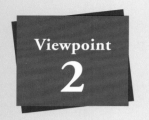

Viewpoint

2

The AIDS Epidemic Remains a Serious Threat

Lorinda Bullock

"HIV/AIDS remains one of the largest global health threats."

Despite medical advances that allow those infected with HIV to live longer, the AIDS epidemic continues to ravage the globe, reports Lorinda Bullock in the following article. There is still no cure for AIDS and no vaccine that prevents HIV infection—and the virus continues to spread in the United States and in developing nations, she points out. Improved education and prevention efforts are still needed to help reduce transmission rates, and more funding is needed to develop an AIDS vaccine. Bullock is an associate editor for Elsevier Global Medical News, an online media company.

AS YOU READ, CONSIDER THE FOLLOWING QUESTIONS:

1. In what year was the AIDS virus discovered?
2. According to Jeffrey S. Crowley, quoted by the author, how many new HIV infections are reported in the United States each year?
3. Which actions can help reduce HIV transmission rates in developing countries, according to Bullock?

Lorinda Bullock, "25 Years Later, HIV/AIDS Still an Epidemic," *Internal Medicine News,* vol. 42, no. 11, June 1, 2009, pp. 14–15. Copyright © 2009 by *Internal Medicine News.* Reproduced by permission.

The two researchers credited with discovering HIV in 1984, Dr. Robert C. Gallo and Dr. Luc A. Montagnier, came together in a "Global Call to Action" to remind the world on the 25th anniversary of their discovery that HIV/AIDS remains one of the largest global health threats.

Despite advances in treatment that allow people with the virus to live longer, "we are still facing an epidemic. There is no cure, no vaccine. The virus is spreading in developing countries," Dr. Montagnier, president of the World Foundation for AIDS Research and Prevention, reminded the public at a media gathering. He stressed that education about HIV/AIDS prevention remains paramount—comparing the disease with the 2009-H1N1 flu that has dominated recent media coverage. "It is transmissible, not contagious like the 'swine flu,'" he said.

Doctors Luc Montagnier, left, and Robert C. Gallo discovered the AIDS virus in 1984. Twenty-five years later, they say that AIDS remains one of the greatest global health threats.

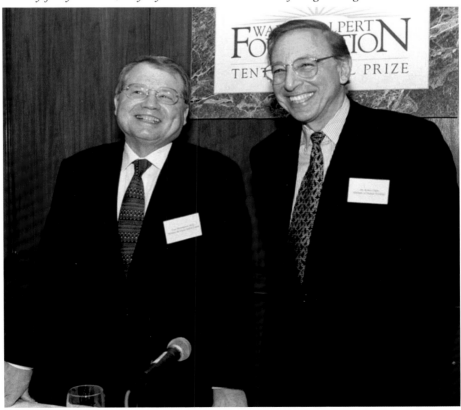

The Enormity of the Epidemic

Dr. Gallo, director of the Institute of Human Virology at the University of Maryland, Baltimore, said the 25th anniversary "is a good time for a reminder. It's not to make criticisms but to make suggestions" about the enormity of the HIV/AIDS epidemic that continues to ravage the globe. The rate is particularly high not only in Africa but also in the United States, where blacks and Hispanics are infected in large numbers.

> **FAST FACT**
>
> According to the Joint United Nations Programme on HIV/AIDS, 60 million people have been infected with HIV and 25 million have died of HIV-related causes since the start of the AIDS epidemic.

The groundbreaking researchers published articles in the May 4, 1984, edition of *Science* that led to the development of the HIV blood test, diagnostic use of which helped to control the pandemic.

Jeffrey S. Crowley, director of the White House Office of National AIDS Policy, said that the [Barack] Obama Administration is working to lower rates of infection, to improve care for people living with the disease, and to find ways to address the health disparities in target populations.

"The president wants to continue America's commitment to the HIV/AIDS epidemic global leadership . . . but he also wants us to solve the domestic HIV/AIDS epidemic," he added.

A Global Call to Action

Mr. Crowley said Americans should not think that HIV/AIDS infection rates have slowed, considering the more than 56,000 new infections being reported in the United States each year.

Key goals of the "Global Call to Action" include:

- Greater investment in medical infrastructure and educational outreach programs in the most-affected U.S. communities.
- Development of HIV/AIDS treatment and control programs with institutions in developing countries. For example, programs that promote better nutrition, which contributes to a healthy immune

system, can help reduce transmission rates and improve the quality of life for infected patients, Dr. Montagnier said.

- Cultivation of young scientists in the field of human virology. "We see less, particularly from the United States. Surely MD's [medical doctors] are not going into research like they did when I was a young man," Dr. Gallo said. More researchers in this field are coming from Eastern Europe, China, and India, he said.
- Enhancement of HIV/AIDS education and prevention, especially in highly affected countries.
- Commitment to the prevention of mother-to-child HIV transmission.

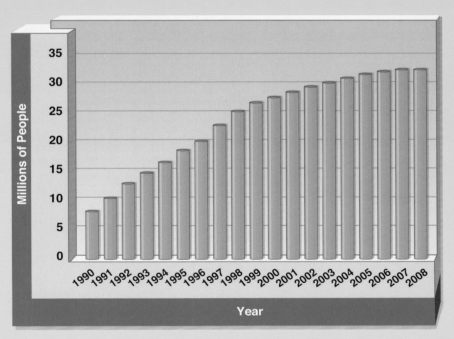

Worldwide HIV Statistics

The number of people living with HIV has risen from around 8 million in 1990 to 33 million in 2008 and is still growing.

- Support for cutting-edge research for vaccines. Dr. Gallo said he believed that "a more major vaccine effort could have been initiated earlier," but he noted that the National Institutes of Health, the Gates Foundation, and others currently are working very hard in vaccine development to make up for lost time.

More Research Is Needed

Although some research out of the University of Pennsylvania, Philadelphia, has been promising, involving the removal of a special receptor with HIV cells and infusing stem cells back together, he noted that such ongoing research is "immensely expensive."

Better therapies would be those that mitigate side effects and treatment resistance, he said, urging pharmaceutical companies to invest in vaccine research.

"We are not dead in AIDS research. There are still new discoveries to be made," Dr. Montagnier said.

EVALUATING THE AUTHORS' ARGUMENTS:

In this viewpoint Lorinda Bullock highlights the main points discussed at a meeting of AIDS researchers. These researchers maintain that advances in the treatment of AIDS should not lull people into thinking that HIV infection rates have slowed. Do you think this contradicts the main point of the preceding selection by the *Global Agenda*? Explain.

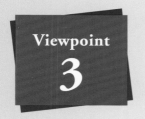

In Developing Countries, Other Public Health Problems Are a Greater Threat Than AIDS

"Many millions . . . die of malnutrition, pneumonia, motor vehicle accidents and other largely preventable, if not headline-grabbing, conditions."

Daniel Halperin

Daniel Halperin, a senior research scientist at the Harvard School of Public Health, formerly served as an HIV prevention adviser for the United States Agency for International Development. In this selection Halperin argues that the AIDS epidemic is serious but needs to be put into perspective. In many African nations, for example, diarrhea, malnutrition, and poor prenatal care are greater threats to public health than HIV is. Because the fight against AIDS is popular, it receives billions in funding while the more common and easily treatable diseases are ignored. Halperin implores donors in wealthy countries to reexamine their global health priorities.

AS YOU READ, CONSIDER THE FOLLOWING QUESTIONS:
1. How much did the United States spend on AIDS programs in Africa in 2007, according to Halperin?
2. What are the adult HIV rates in the majority of African nations, according to the author?
3. In Halperin's view, what are the biggest public health threats in Senegal?

Although the United Nations recently lowered its global H.I.V. estimates, as many as 33 million people worldwide are still living with the AIDS virus [as of January 2008]. This pandemic requires continued attention; preventing further deaths and orphans remains imperative. But the well-meaning promises of some presidential candidates to outdo even President [George W.] Bush's proposal to nearly double American foreign assistance to fight AIDS strike me, an H.I.V.-AIDS specialist for 15 years, as missing the mark.

Some have criticized Mr. Bush for requesting "only" $30 billion for the next five years for AIDS and related problems, with the leading Democratic candidates having pledged to commit at least $50 billion if they are elected. Yet even the current $15 billion in spending represents an unprecedented amount of money aimed mainly at a single disease.

Meanwhile, many other public health needs in developing countries are being ignored. The fact is, spending $50 billion or more on foreign health assistance does make sense, but only if it is not limited to H.I.V.-AIDS programs.

A Huge Imbalance

Last year [2007], for instance, as the United States spent almost $3 billion on AIDS programs in Africa, it invested only about $30 million in traditional safe-water projects. This nearly 100-to-1 imbalance is disastrously inequitable—especially considering that in Africa H.I.V. tends to be most prevalent in the relatively wealthiest and most developed countries. Most African nations have stable adult H.I.V. rates of 3 percent or less.

Many millions of African children and adults die of malnutrition, pneumonia, motor vehicle accidents and other largely preventable, if not headline-grabbing, conditions. One-fifth of all global deaths from diarrhea occur in just three African countries—Congo, Ethiopia and Nigeria—that have relatively low H.I.V. prevalence. Yet this condition, which is not particularly difficult to cure or prevent, gets scant attention from the donors that invest nearly $1 billion annually on AIDS programs in those countries.

Misguided Priorities

I was struck by this discrepancy between Western donors' priorities and the real needs of Africans last month [December 2007], during my most recent trip to Africa. In Senegal, H.I.V. rates remain under 1 percent in adults, partly due to that country's early adoption of enlightened policies toward prostitution and other risky practices, in addition to universal male circumcision, which limits the heterosexual spread of H.I.V. Rates of tuberculosis, now another favored disease of international donors, are also relatively low in Senegal, and I learned

AIDS patients languish at a clinic in Africa. In many African countries diarrhea, malnutrition, and poor prenatal care are bigger threats to public health than AIDS.

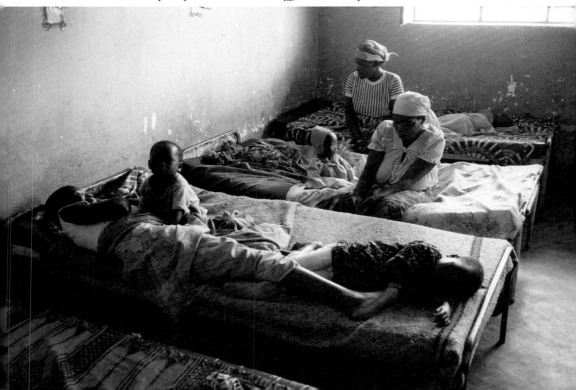

that even malaria, the donors third major concern, is not quite as rampant as was assumed, with new testing finding that many fevers aren't actually caused by the disease.

Meanwhile, the stench of sewage permeates the crowded outskirts of Dakar, Senegal's capital. There, as in many other parts of West Africa and the developing world, inadequate access to safe water results in devastating diarrheal diseases. Shortages of food and basic health services like vaccinations, prenatal care and family planning contribute to large family size and high child and maternal mortality. Major donors like the President's Emergency Plan for AIDS Relief, known as PEPFAR, and the Global Fund to Fight AIDS, Tuberculosis and Malaria have not directly addressed such basic health issues. The Global Fund's director, Michel Kazatchkine, has acknowledged, "We are not a global fund that funds local health."

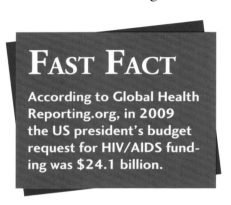

FAST FACT

According to Global Health Reporting.org, in 2009 the US president's budget request for HIV/AIDS funding was $24.1 billion.

Botswana, which has the world's most lucrative diamond industry and is the second-wealthiest country per capita in sub-Saharan Africa, is nowhere near as burdened as Senegal with basic public health problems. But as one of a dozen PEPFAR "focus" countries in Africa, this year it will receive about $300 million to fight AIDS—in addition to the hundreds of millions already granted by drug companies, private foundations and other donors. While in that sparsely populated country last month, I learned that much of its AIDS money remains unspent, as even its state-of-the-art H.I.V. clinics cannot absorb such a large influx of cash.

More Common Illnesses Are Ignored

As the United States Agency for International Development's H.I.V. prevention adviser in southern Africa in 2005 and 2006, I visited villages in poor countries like Lesotho, where clinics could not afford to stock basic medicines but often maintained an inventory of expensive AIDS drugs and sophisticated monitoring equipment for their H.I.V.

patients. H.I.V.-infected children are offered exemplary treatment, while children suffering from much simpler-to-treat diseases are left untreated, sometimes to die.

In Africa, there's another crisis exacerbated by the rigid focus on AIDS: The best health practitioners have abandoned lower-paying positions in family planning, immunization and other basic health areas in order to work for donor-financed H.I.V. programs.

The AIDS experience has demonstrated that poor countries can make complex treatments accessible to many people. Regimens that are much simpler to administer than anti-retroviral drugs—like anti-biotics for respiratory illnesses, oral rehydration for diarrhea, immu-nizations and contraception—could also be made widely available. But as there isn't a "global fund" for safe water, child survival and family planning, countries like Senegal—and even poorer ones—cannot directly tackle their real problems without pegging them to the big three diseases.

Addressing Real-World Needs

To their credit, some AIDS advocates are calling for a broader approach to international health programs. Among the presiden-tial candidates, Senator Barack Obama, for example, proposes to go beyond spending for AIDS, tuberculosis and malaria, highlight-ing the need to also strengthen basic health systems. And recent-ly, Mr. Bush's plan, along with the Global Fund, has become somewhat more flexible in supporting other health issues linked to H.I.V.—though this will be of little use to people, especially outside the "focus" countries, who are dying of common illnesses like diarrhea.

But it is also important, especially for the United States, the world's largest donor, to re-examine the epidemiological and moral foundations of its global health priorities. With 10 million children and a half million mothers in developing countries dying annu-ally of largely preventable conditions, should we mutiply AIDS spending while giving only a pittance for initiatives like safe-water projects?

If one were to ask the people of virtually any African village (outside some 10 countries devastated by AIDS) what their greatest concerns are, the answer would undoubtedly be the less sensational but more ubiquitous ravages of hunger, dirty water and environmental devastation. The real-world needs of Africans struggling to survive should not continue to be subsumed by the favorite causes du jour [of the day] of well-meaning yet often uninformed Western donors.

EVALUATING THE AUTHOR'S ARGUMENTS:

Daniel Halperin contends that global health advocates have focused so much on combating AIDS that other more common and simpler-to-treat diseases are being ignored. He believes that some of the funding earmarked for AIDS should instead be used to treat malnutrition, diarrhea, pneumonia, and other illnesses. What evidence does he use to support his argument? Is his evidence convincing? Explain.

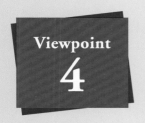

AIDS Is the Greatest Health Threat in Some Nations

"The HIV/ AIDS pandemic remains a real threat in the developing world."

The Post-Standard **Editorial Board**

Some experts argue that since the AIDS epidemic has peaked, some of the funding devoted to combating HIV should be used for fighting other global health problems instead. In the upcoming selection the editors of a Syracuse, New York, daily newspaper, *The Post-Standard,* disagree with this view. In many sub-Saharan African nations, AIDS remains the leading cause of death, the authors point out. There are many who do not yet know they are infected with HIV, as well as a growing number of AIDS orphans. Resources for AIDS prevention and treatment should remain a priority, the editors conclude.

AS YOU READ, CONSIDER THE FOLLOWING QUESTIONS:
1. How many people die daily from the effects of the AIDS virus, according to this viewpoint?
2. According to the authors, what is the estimated number of AIDS orphans in Nigeria?
3. How much higher is the HIV infection rate in US prisons compared to the nonprison population?

I s this the beginning of the "post-AIDS era"? If so, that would be something to celebrate. Has the virus that held the world hostage during the 1980s and 1990s been defeated?

Jeremy Shiffman, associate professor of public administration at Syracuse University's Maxwell School, recently [in 2008] told the Associated Press: "AIDS is a terrible humanitarian tragedy, but it's just one of many terrible humanitarian tragedies."

Professor Shiffman makes a good point. A range of ills plagues much of the developing world—from malaria and river blindness to diarrhea and iodine deficiency. The needs of children and others facing these challenges are just as compelling as those of people with HIV/AIDS.

Yet others go further, arguing that the AIDS juggernaut is too big and too costly, and that resources should be diverted to other health care battles.

Not so fast.

> **FAST FACT**
>
> The Joint United Nations Programme on HIV/AIDS reports that for every two people starting HIV treatment, another five are newly infected.

A Relentless Toll

Even while the number of infections in the United States and other developed nations peaked in the 1990s; even as medical breakthroughs can make HIV/AIDS a chronic condition rather than a death sentence, there are exceptions.

Like Africa. HIV/AIDS remains the leading cause of death south of the Sahara, home to the majority of the 33 million people worldwide

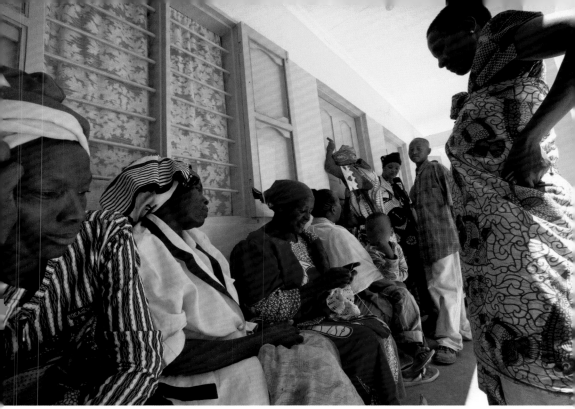

Women and men wait to be tested outside an HIV clinic in Tanzania. In many sub-Saharan African countries, AIDS remains the leading cause of death.

believed to be living with HIV/AIDS—and the 5,500 people dying each day from the effects of the virus. Most of those who carry the virus still don't know it, since they haven't been tested.

About 3 million people receive life-saving antiretroviral AIDS medications. But the toll grows relentlessly. In Nigeria alone, there are an estimated 930,000 "AIDS orphans."

A Persistent Problem

Closer to home, the infection numbers are smaller, but they persist. In 2006, the latest year on record, 56,300 Americans were newly infected with HIV—men, women, minorities, drug users, youths, seniors, prison inmates, veterans.

In New York state, 116,384 people were living with HIV/AIDS last December [2007]—4,376 of them infected that year. The 11-county Central/Northern New York region had 1,685 active HIV/AIDS cases.

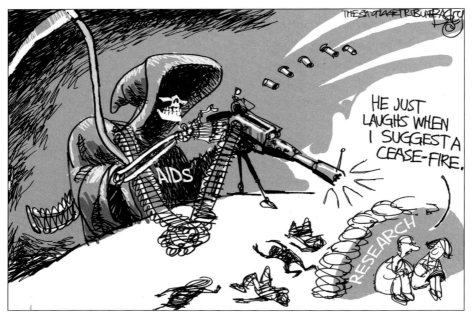

"AIDS Cease-Fire," cartoon by Pat Bagley, *Salt Lake Tribune,* August 15, 2006, PoliticalCartoons.com. Copyright © 2006 by Pat Bagley and CagleCartoons.com. All rights reserved.

There are several new and promising initiatives, both at home and abroad. Among them:

The "One Million Tests" campaign, conducted the week before World AIDS Day Dec. 1 [2008], aims to ramp up HIV testing and treatment around the world—a key to halting the pandemic.

In New York City, the world's first AIDS vaccine facility is setting up shop. An effective vaccine is another key to stopping AIDS in its tracks.

A measure making its way through Congress would combat HIV/ AIDS in U.S. prisons, where the infection rate is three times that of the general population.

The Threat Remains

To his credit, President [George W.] Bush ramped up the U.S. com- mitment to the global AIDS effort. But that effort is faltering as the administration winds down. President-elect [Barack] Obama has pledged to redouble his predecessor's commitment—though budget pressures are sure to be intense.

It's a promise worth keeping. The HIV/AIDS pandemic remains a real threat in the developing world. Even in Central New York, where the threat is more manageable, there is a long way to go.

EVALUATING THE AUTHORS' ARGUMENTS:

The Post-Standard maintains that since AIDS remains a devastating epidemic, resources for fighting HIV should not be diverted to other global health-care battles. In the preceding selection, Daniel Halperin argues that global assistance focuses too much on AIDS and neglects other pressing health challenges. With which viewpoint do you most strongly agree? Why?

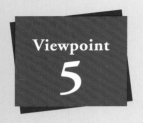

Access to AIDS Treatment Has Improved

"The fact that more people than ever are on treatment is evidence that our efforts to combat HIV/AIDS are paying off."

amfAR, The Foundation for AIDS Research

In the following article amfAR, The Foundation for AIDS Research reports that there has been a significant increase in the number of people in poorer countries receiving treatment for HIV infection. This data reveals that access to AIDS testing, medication, and counseling has greatly improved, the authors point out. There is still plenty of room for progress, however, because the rates of testing and counseling among high-risk groups remain distressingly low. AmfAR, The Foundation for AIDS Research is a nonprofit organization dedicated to supporting AIDS research and HIV prevention.

AS YOU READ, CONSIDER THE FOLLOWING QUESTIONS:

1. At the end of 2008, what percentage of HIV-positive people in poorer nations were able to receive treatment, according to this report?
2. What percentage of HIV-positive pregnant women living in poorer nations received antiretroviral drugs in 2007? In 2008?
3. According to the author, what groups are at high risk for HIV infection?

Iwnternational efforts to expand access to HIV treatment have resulted in a tenfold increase during the past five years in the number of people in low- and middle-income countries receiving antiretroviral treatment (ART), according to a report recently released [as of October 2009] by WHO, UNAIDS, and UNICEF [international aid organizations]. HIV testing and counseling are also more widely available, with a 35 percent increase over 2007 in the number of health facilities providing testing.

"The fact that more people than ever are on treatment is evidence that our efforts to combat HIV/AIDS are paying off," said amfAR [Foundation for AIDS Research] CEO Kevin Robert Frost. "We need

Antiretroviral drugs are prepared for distribution to HIV patients in Jakarta, Indonesia. The number of people in low- to middle-income countries receiving antiretroviral treatment increased tenfold from 2005 to 2009.

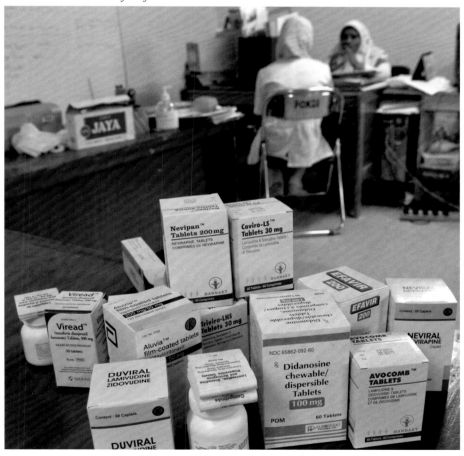

to continue to invest in treatment, prevention, and care to ensure that all people who need them can receive the services they deserve."

More People Are Receiving Treatment

According to the report, at the end of 2008 approximately 42 percent of HIV-positive people in need of treatment in low- and middle-income countries were receiving it—an increase of 36 percent over 2007. The same period saw a dramatic increase (80 percent) in the number of health facilities that provide ART to children under 15, and 39 percent more children were receiving ART.

Services for pregnant women—including HIV testing, counseling, and treatment—also expanded in 2008; nearly half (45 percent) of HIV-positive pregnant women received ART to prevent transmission to their infants, compared with 35 percent in 2007. New prevention interventions such as male circumcision were also scaled up in 2008, most notably in sub-Saharan Africa, where HIV is largely spread through heterosexual transmission and rates of male circumcision are low.

Remaining Obstacles to Access

Despite these gains, the report also revealed some significant obstacles to universal access—most discouraging the fact that the number of new infections continues to outpace the number of people receiving treatment. Although more people are being tested for HIV, the majority of those living with the virus still remain unaware of their status. Rates of testing and counseling remain particularly low among high-risk groups, including injection drug users (23 percent), men who have sex with men, or MSM (30 percent), and sex workers (38 percent).

The report highlighted the need for enhanced prevention efforts for these groups, particularly injection drug users, most of whom do not have access to syringe exchange programs and other harm reduc-

Progress	December 2007	December 2008
Number of adults and children receiving antiretroviral therapy	2,970,000	4,030,000
Antiretroviral therapy coverage among adults and children	33%	42%
Number of children younger than 15 years in need of receiving antiretroviral therapy	198,000	275,700
Percentage of pregnant women living with HIV and receiving antiretroviral drugs to prevent mother-to-child transmission	35%	45%

Taken from: American Foundation for AIDS Research (amfAR), *Toward Universal Access, Progress Report 2009,* Executive Summary. (WHO, UNAIDS, UNICEF).

tion services. The median rate of condom use among surveyed MSM was approximately 60 percent, but rates varied widely, and many countries still do not have sufficient data on the spread of the epidemic among this vulnerable population. Tuberculosis [TB] remains another concern, as ART coverage for people living with both HIV and TB remains very low.

EVALUATING THE AUTHORS' ARGUMENTS:

This selection cites Kevin Robert Frost, the CEO of amfAR, The Foundation for AIDS Research, who claims that the increase in the number of people receiving antiretroviral drugs proves that efforts to combat AIDS are "paying off." Given what you have read elsewhere in this text, do you agree or disagree with Frost's assertion? Why or why not?

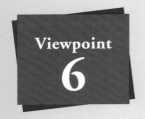
Stigma and Misconceptions About AIDS Remain

"A significant share of the public . . . harbors misconceptions about prevention and treatment of HIV/AIDS."

The Henry J. Kaiser Family Foundation

Even though the Centers for Disease Control and Prevention recently announced that the US HIV epidemic is larger than previously thought, Americans have less of a sense of urgency about AIDS, reports The Kaiser Family Foundation in the following viewpoint. Young adults and those who are in high-risk groups are less concerned about the possibility that they may become infected, and the rate of AIDS testing has not increased over the past decade. Moreover, significant percentages of Americans are still unclear about how HIV is transmitted and how HIV infection can be prevented. The Kaiser Family Foundation is a nonprofit private operating foundation, based in Menlo Park, California.

AS YOU READ, CONSIDER THE FOLLOWING QUESTIONS:
1. What percentage of young adults reported being tested for HIV in the past year, according to The Kaiser Family Foundation?
2. What fraction of Americans claims to have donated money to an AIDS-related charity, according to the author?
3. What percentage of the public admits to being uncomfortable about having their food prepared by someone infected with HIV?

Washington, DC—Less than a year after the Centers for Disease Control and Prevention (CDC) recalculated the size of the HIV/AIDS epidemic and announced that there were 40 percent more new HIV infections each year than previously believed, a new survey by the Kaiser Family Foundation finds that Americans' sense of urgency about HIV/AIDS as a national health problem has fallen dramatically and their concern about HIV as a personal risk has also declined, even among some groups at higher risk.

Key findings of the survey include:

- The share of Americans naming HIV/AIDS as the most urgent health problem facing the nation dropped precipitously from 44 percent in 1995 to 17 percent in 2006 and to six percent now.
- CDC estimates that HIV rates are seven times higher among African Americans and three times higher among Latinos compared to whites. While these groups are more likely than whites to see HIV/AIDS as an urgent problem, fewer say it is a "more urgent" problem for their community now than in 2006 (declining from 23% to 17% of all adults, 49% to 40% of African Americans, and 46% to 35% of Latinos).
- The share of those ages 18–29 who say they are personally very concerned about becoming infected with HIV declined from 30 percent in 1997 to 17 percent today; personal concern among young African Americans declined from 54 percent to 40 percent over the same time period.
- More than half (53%) of non-elderly adults say they have been tested for HIV, including 19 percent who say they were tested in

the past year. Testing is most common among adults under the age of 30, with three in ten young adults and nearly half (47%) of young African Americans reporting having been tested in the past year. However, reported testing rates for all these groups have not changed much in the past decade.

"Many indicators of urgency and concern are moving in the wrong direction, including for higher risk groups," said Kaiser President and CEO Drew Altman. "The survey underscores the need for a new focus on domestic HIV," he added.

At a time when there have been calls for increased attention to the domestic HIV/AIDS crisis including the recent [Barack] Obama administration announcement of the five year public awareness campaign, Act Against AIDS, the survey also finds public support for more spending.

Half of the public thinks that the federal government is spending too little on domestic HIV/AIDS, while just five percent say it spends too much. More than a third (36%) of Americans say they have personally donated money to an HIV/AIDS-related charity, including nearly half (45%) of African Americans, and there is confidence that new efforts in prevention will make a difference.

While down somewhat from 2006, public support for continued or increased government spending on HIV/AIDS is notable considering the current economic recession and a decline in reported visibility of the domestic epidemic. The share saying they have heard, seen, or read "a lot" or "some" about the problem of HIV/AIDS in the U.S. in the past year declined from 70 percent in 2004 to 45 percent in 2009, and the share that saw "a lot" was cut in half for not only the general public, but also among African Americans and Latinos.

Despite a polarizing debate in recent years about such issues as abstinence and condoms, six in ten Americans believe that spending more money on HIV prevention in the U.S. will lead to meaningful progress, and about half believe the same about spending on treatment.

Some Signs of Progress, but Misconceptions and Stigma Remain

The survey indicates some signs that HIV/AIDS in the U.S. may carry less stigma than in the past. For instance, there has been a slow and

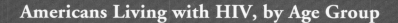

Americans Living with HIV, by Age Group

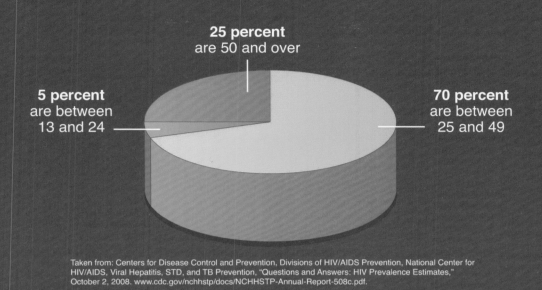

25 percent
are 50 and over

5 percent
are between
13 and 24

70 percent
are between
25 and 49

Taken from: Centers for Disease Control and Prevention, Divisions of HIV/AIDS Prevention, National Center for HIV/AIDS, Viral Hepatitis, STD, and TB Prevention, "Questions and Answers: HIV Prevalence Estimates," October 2, 2008. www.cdc.gov/nchhstp/docs/NCHHSTP-Annual-Report-508c.pdf.

steady increase since the late 1990s in the share of people who say they would be very comfortable with a coworker who has HIV/AIDS (44% now, up from 32% in 1997). However, stigmatizing attitudes towards people with HIV have not gone away; fully half (51%) of the public says they would be uncomfortable having their food prepared by someone who is HIV positive.

Misconceptions may be a factor in stigma, and several remain when it comes to correct information about HIV transmission. One-third (34%) of Americans incorrectly believe or are unsure whether HIV can be transmitted by one of the following actions: sharing a drinking glass (27%), touching a toilet seat (17%), or swimming in a pool with an HIV positive person (14%).

Confusion about HIV transmission may contribute to discomfort around those who are HIV positive. People who harbor misconceptions about transmission are more likely to say they would be uncomfortable working with someone with HIV (43% versus 13% who correctly answered questions about transmission) and more likely to be uncomfortable having their food prepared by an HIV positive person (71% compared to 40%).

A significant share of the public also harbors misconceptions about prevention and treatment of HIV/AIDS. Nearly one in five (18%) do not know there is no cure for AIDS and about one-quarter (27%) believe or are unsure whether former professional basketball player Magic Johnson has been cured of AIDS. Additionally, a quarter (24%) believe or are unsure whether there is a vaccine available to prevent HIV infection. Many of these misconceptions are more common in the African American community, including that Magic Johnson has been cured (37% of African Americans think he has been cured or are unsure), that there is a vaccine available to prevent infection (36%), and that there are drugs available that can cure HIV and AIDS (30%).

Methodology

The survey was designed and analyzed by public opinion researchers at the Kaiser Family Foundation and was conducted January 26 through March 8, 2009, among a nationally representative random sample of 2,554 adults ages 18 and older. Telephone interviews conducted by landline (N=1,951) and cell phone (N=603, including 214 who had no landline telephone) were carried out in English and Spanish. The survey includes oversamples of African American and Latino respondents as well as respondents ages 18-29. Results for all groups have been weighted to reflect their actual distribution in the nation. The margin of sampling error for the overall survey is plus or minus 3 percentage points, for whites it is plus or minus 4 percentage points, for African Americans it is plus or minus 5 percentage points, and for Latinos it is plus or minus 6 percentage points. For results based on other subgroups, the margin of sampling error may be higher.

The full question wording, results, charts and a brief on the poll can be viewed online.

EVALUATING THE AUTHOR'S ARGUMENTS:

This selection from The Kaiser Family Foundation includes surveys showing that many people still harbor misconceptions about how HIV is transmitted. What are these misconceptions? Do you find these misconceptions to be common among the people you know? Explain.

Chapter 2

How Can the Spread of AIDS Be Controlled?

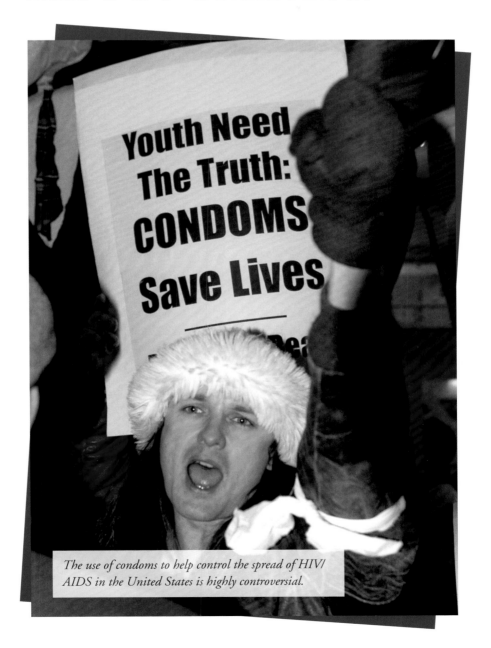

The use of condoms to help control the spread of HIV/ AIDS in the United States is highly controversial.

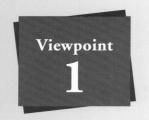

Viewpoint

1

Access to Testing and Treatment Can Stop the Spread of AIDS

"Anti-retroviral drugs are extraordinarily successful at containing the virus in patients who are already infected."

Mark Henderson

The spread of HIV around the globe and the lack of a cure or a vaccine for AIDS is one of science's great failures, notes *The Times* (London) science editor Mark Henderson in the following viewpoint. However, antiretroviral drugs have proved to be very successful in controlling the virus in those who are already infected. Universal testing and treatment programs—if combined with education and behavioral changes—could be the key to preventing the spread of AIDS, Henderson concludes.

AS YOU READ, CONSIDER THE FOLLOWING QUESTIONS:
1. What year was HIV identified as the virus that causes AIDS?
2. According to Henderson, how might AIDS drugs eventually do much of the work of a vaccine?
3. What needs to be done before universal testing and treatment programs are implemented, in the author's view?

The global extent of the HIV pandemic is one of the great failures of modern science. While the identity of the virus that causes Aids has been known since 1983, and its discoverers have won the Nobel Prize for Medicine, it has not yet proved possible to stop it from spreading.

Vaccine research has hit dead end after dead end, as HIV's diabolical ability to mutate has confounded every promising candidate, and vaginal microbicides designed to prevent transmission have also disappointed.

Public health interventions such as condoms have worked, but require behaviour changes that can be difficult to achieve.

Students attend an HIV/AIDS education class in Indonesia. Education and behavioral changes combined with testing and treatment may be able to prevent the spread of AIDS.

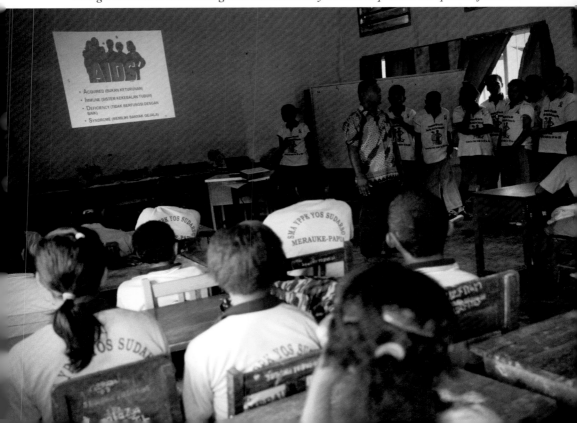

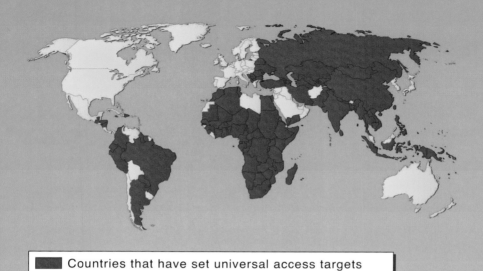

Nations Commited to the Goal of Providing Universal Access to HIV Treatment

Countries that have set universal access targets
Countries that have not set universal access targets

Taken from: UNAIDS.org, July 23, 2009. www.unaids.org/en/KnowledgeCenter/HIVData/mapping_progress.asp.

One Major Success

This failure, however, has been matched with one great triumph: Anti-retroviral drugs are extraordinarily successful at containing the virus in patients who are already infected.

Where HIV was once seen as a death sentence, it is now regarded as a chronic condition with which people can live for decades.

There is now a good chance that this success can be exploited to prevent the spread of HIV.

As drugs reduce the amount of virus in the body, they make carriers less infectious, so they have the potential to do much of the job of a vaccine.

The universal testing and treatment programme proposed by [epidemiologist] Brian Williams[1] has a good chance of delivering a steep

---

1. In 2009 Brain Williams and his colleagues at the World Health Organization proposed a program in which any adult over the age of 15 would be tested annually for HIV. Those who tested positive would then immediately begin treatment with antiretroviral drugs.

change in HIV prevention, particularly if combined with safe sex education and male circumcision.

Remaining Hurdles

Several important hurdles remain, however. First, the approach must be rigorously analysed in randomised trials, to confirm that it can actually work in African settings.

We need to know whether people will accept mass testing, and whether those who test positive will complete their treatment: Poor compliance can build drug-resistance and make the problem worse.

There is also the matter of cost. While containing Aids would certainly pay for itself in the long run, significant up-front investment will be needed.

The sums involved are large, but not that large: Dr Williams compared the estimated $3billion needed for South Africa with the $30[billion] cost of the Iraq troop surge.

They are certainly not beyond the combined means of Western and African governments, and philanthropic organisations such as the Bill & Melinda Gates Foundation.

To engage these resources, though, firm evidence of efficacy will be needed. That is why the trials that start soon in South Africa[2] are so important.

2. In mid-2010 South Africa began a widespread campaign to encourage HIV counseling and testing. The country hopes to test 15 million of its 47 million residents by June 2011.

EVALUATING THE AUTHORS' ARGUMENTS:

Mark Henderson maintains that universal access to anti-retroviral drugs could play a major role in preventing the spread of HIV. Considering the other preventative strategies that are discussed in this volume, do you agree? Why or why not? Use evidence from the text in explaining your answer.

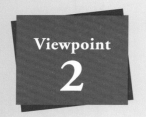
Access to Testing and Treatment Will Not Stop the Spread of AIDS

Elizabeth Pisani

"[Hailing] expanded HIV treatment in Africa as the new answer to prevention [is] a triumph of optimism over common sense."

The notion that providing universal access to HIV testing and treatment will eventually stop the spread of AIDS is dangerously misguided, argues Elizabeth Pisani in the following viewpoint. She states that, for one thing, HIV spreads more rapidly right after people have been infected—before they have been tested and know they are carrying the virus. Furthermore, condom use has decreased because the current effectiveness of antiretroviral drugs has created a false sense of security. New infections are actually on the rise in at-risk groups, Pisani points out. It is very risky to focus on expanded treatment of HIV while neglecting education and prevention efforts, she concludes. Pisani, an epidemiologist and author, directs Ternyata Ltd., a public health consultancy in London, England.

I t's been a bad few months for HIV prevention. We've learned that our best candidates for vaccines and virus-killing microbicides don't work. Now we're clutching at another straw: maybe we can treat our way out of the HIV epidemic.

At an HIV research meeting this week [in February 2010], boffins [scientists] from the World Health Organisation revived a mathematical model that shows that if we test everyone in Africa for HIV once a year and give everyone who tests positive expensive drugs right away and for the rest of their lives, we'll wipe out new HIV infections within seven years. That's because HIV is passed on most easily when there's lots of virus in the infected person's blood and body fluids. Antiretroviral medicines cut the "viral load" (the amount of virus in the body), so they make it more difficult to pass on HIV. Ergo, more treatment means fewer new infections.

> **FAST FACT**
>
> According to the independent news organization Kaisernetwork.org, 150 million condoms are needed each year in Uganda, but less than 40 million were provided in 2005.

Not So Fast

Sadly, it's not that simple. For one thing, HIV is most infectious in the few months after a person is first infected. Even if everyone got tested annually, we'd miss most of these new infections. Second, people's viral load spikes upwards if they get another sexually transmitted infection (STI), or if they stop taking their medicine because the

The Four Stages of HIV/AIDS

1. Primary HIV infection: Lasts from a few weeks to six months

- possible flu-like symptoms
- swollen lymph nodes
- may have no symptoms

2. Asymptomatic HIV: Lasts ten or more years

- usually symptom-free, but HIV is reproducing constantly in the body
- mild weight loss
- respiratory infections
- fungal nail infections
- recurring mouth sores

3. Symptomatic HIV: Length of this stage varies

- at first symptoms are mild, but they grow more severe
- chronic diarrhea
- persistent fever
- bacterial infections
- anemia
- moderate to severe weight loss
- cancers
- shingles
- tuberculosis

4. AIDS: Length of this stage varies

- recurrent severe pneumonia
- parasitic diseases
- meningitis
- blood poisoning
- lymphoma
- Kaposi's sarcoma
- HIV wasting syndrome with severe weight loss

Taken from: Jamie Robertson, "WHO Clinical Staging for HIV Infection," January 7, 2009. www.suite101.com.

clinic runs out of stock, the meds make them feel sick, or they went on a three-day bender and forgot their pills. Interrupting treatment also allows the virus to develop resistance to drugs, and that leads to more spikes in viral load. Most importantly, antiretrovirals keep you alive and well enough to be out there meeting new sex partners. That's a good thing, obviously, but it also means that people who have HIV are going to have more chances to pass it on during those times when their viral load is spiky.

There's more. In countries like the UK [United Kingdom] where treatment has been available for over a decade, Aids has virtually disappeared. HIV, unfortunately, has not. A few years after antiretrovirals became widely available, new infections among gay men in the UK began to rise. We've seen the same thing in Australia, the United States and practically everywhere else we have data. One reason for that is that gay men use condoms less now than they did when HIV = Aids = a horrible death. Now, though, HIV = a pill every day. Boring, but not the end of the world, unless you're the taxpayer picking up the tab for it or the epidemiologist worrying that drug-resistant strains of HIV will reignite Aids.

Dangerous Optimism

On top of that, many people assume that if the person they're having sex with is infected, they'll be on meds and so not very infectious. Which may be true if they're not in that early peak of infectiousness, have taken all their pills diligently, and don't have another STI. Though since condom use is dropping across the board, other STI rates are soaring. In short, more people living with HIV, combined with more unprotected sex is outweighing the effects of lower viral load in places where the population is well informed, HIV testing is actively promoted, and treatment has been free and universally available. But in Africa it will be different.

Our computer model assumes every African will get tested for HIV every year, everyone who tests positive will start taking antiretrovirals immediately and 98 out of 100 will never miss a dose. On top of that, though gay men in rich countries use condoms far less now than they did before we had antiretrovirals, we assume that heterosexuals in Africa are going to use them more once the most visible and frightening face of Aids disappears.

On the strength of this model, which bears as much relation to reality as an MP's [member of Parliament's] expense claim, we are going to hail expanded HIV treatment in Africa as the new answer to prevention. A triumph of optimism over common sense.

Abstinence and Fidelity Slow the Spread of AIDS

Ernest W. Lefever

"The best way to control the HIV virus [is] to encourage abstinence."

In the 1980s the recognition that promiscuity was a main cause of AIDS in Africa led Ugandan president Yoweri Museveni to launch a vigorous abstinence campaign that reduced the spread of HIV in his country during the 1990s. But today, notes Ernest W. Lefever in the following selection, most AIDS-related funding is spent on testing, condom promotion, and drug treatment. Despite the billions of dollars that wealthy nations have given to combat the spread of AIDS, however, HIV remains pandemic in Africa. In Lefever's opinion, a return to programs stressing abstinence and fidelity would better serve African nations. Lefever is a senior fellow at the Ethics and Public Policy Center in Washington, D.C.

AS YOU READ, CONSIDER THE FOLLOWING QUESTIONS:

1. How many people die of AIDS each day in sub-Saharan Africa, according to the author?
2. In Lefever's view, what is the chief cause of AIDS in Africa?
3. Name the three elements of the abstinence campaign that was launched by Ugandan president Yoweri Museveni in the 1980s.

In sub-Saharan Africa an estimated 30 million people have the HIV-AIDS virus. Some 17 million have died so far, and the disease kills 5,000 adults and 1,000 children every day—a rate 20 times that of Western countries. The crisis is especially grievous because it adds millions of victims to those killed by tribal wars and genocide in postcolonial Africa.

To stem the tide of suffering and death, billions of dollars have been given or pledged by the U.S. Government, other wealthy countries, U.N. agencies, and American philanthropists. But the pandemic continues.

The causes of the AIDS-HIV plague in Africa are known, but efforts to prevent transmission, or slow it down, have run into complex problems.

World Bank President Paul Wolfowitz underscored the crisis in sub-Saharan Africa: "Between 1981 and 2002, the number of people living in poverty . . . nearly doubled, from more than 160 million to more than 300 million."

FAST FACT

The United States Agency for International Development reports that in Uganda, HIV prevalence among pregnant women fell from 30 percent in 1990 to about 10 percent in 2001.

Honest News About AIDS

Despite this dire picture, there is a gleam of hope. Ironically, it comes from Uganda, a country that had suffered terribly under its late president [Idi] Amin, who called himself "The Last King of Scotland" and slaughtered millions of his people.

In 1986, there was some honest news about AIDS—a public acknowledgment that its chief cause in Africa was rampant promiscuity, especially by young males who prey on defenseless girls. Years later, in a *Foreign Affairs* article (Jan.–Feb. 2004) on "The Politics of AIDS," Dr. Holly Burkhalter, an AIDS specialist with Physicians for Human Rights, cited evidence of increasing promiscuity in Africa. She quoted Dr. Karl Peltzer of Cape Town [South Africa], who said the widespread pursuit of young women by older men "has led to a disproportionate number of girls becoming infected. Young girls— some under age 5—are often raped by men, purportedly because of a widespread myth that sex with a virgin can cure or prevent AIDS." Such assaults have generated "millions of orphans and street children . . . who are especially vulnerable to rape and to being forced into the commercial sex industry."

Dr. Burkhalter added: "The predators who sustain the forced-sex trade and child rape industry . . . should be punished severely," but this "almost never occurs." She calls for strategies to fight AIDS transmission by forced prostitution and "voluntary sex."

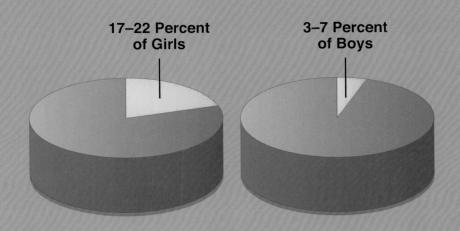

Percentage of Eastern and Southern African Youth Aged 15 to 19 Who Are HIV Positive

17–22 Percent
of Girls

3–7 Percent
of Boys

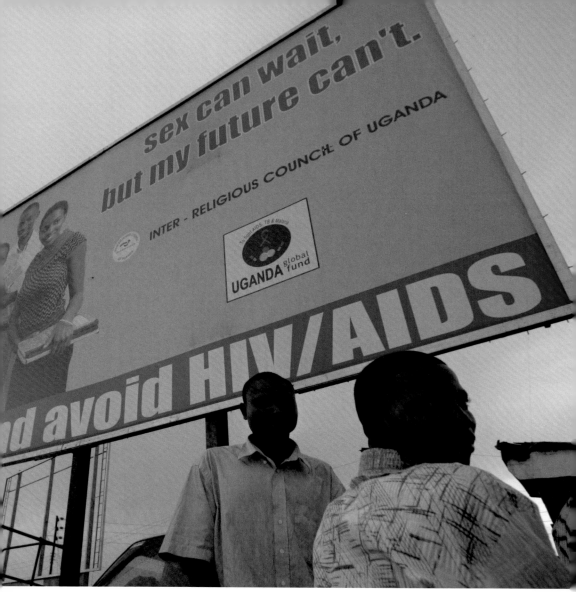

Abstinence programs were started in Uganda in the late 1980s, and they have led to a reduction in HIV infections.

A Gleam of Hope

During the worsening crisis in the mid-1980s, only one African leader seemed to have read the writing on the wall, President Yoweri Museveni of Uganda. Oddly, his awakening was inspired by a brief conversation about AIDS with Fidel Castro at a 1986 conference in Zimbabwe. Castro told Museveni bluntly: "Hey, brother, you have a problem."

Back home, Museveni quickly huddled with his doctors to discuss the issue and consulted several Christian medical missionaries who had already addressed the problem. They agreed that the best way to control the HIV virus was to encourage abstinence. Zeroing in on the root cause, Museveni launched a vigorous three-part campaign promoting abstinence before marriage, fidelity in marriage, and, only then, the use of condoms. Museveni put it bluntly to young males: "No grazing!"

He was criticized by other African leaders and Westerners as naive and moralistic, but his campaign reduced the rate of new AIDS cases from 22 percent in 1992 to 7 percent in 2002, winning plaudits from the World Health Organization. In contrast, most African regimes were in denial about the cause of HIV-AIDS. And foreign donors, attentive to unpopular facts, were reluctant to press the issue and focused more on treatment than prevention.

Fidelity Works Better than Drugs

Rock Star Bono [of the musical group U2] urged America to give a $1 billion grant to combat the scourge in Africa. Since then, most money from wealthy countries has gone to easing the pain of those already infected with HIV or those with full-blown AIDS. This emphasis reflects the earlier American approach to dealing with AIDS, when it was politically incorrect to openly address the fundamental cause of the plague—promiscuity, exacerbated by forceable sex with young girls.

Today in Africa, under the pressure of financial aid and Hollywood hoopla, Uganda's early success in curbing AIDS may be slowing, smothered by ignorance, an unresponsive bureaucracy, and a seemingly endless flow of experimental drugs.

This point is made in a carefully researched article by Craig Timberg of the Washington Post Foreign Service. He writes from Uganda: "Despite [this country's] success story, unmatched elsewhere on this AIDS-ridden continent, no country has entirely replicated Uganda's approach. Most instead have followed the diffuse palette of other remedies pushed by Western doctors—condom promotion, abstinence training, HIV testing, drug treatment, and stigma reduction—while forgoing what research shows worked here: fear and a relentless focus on fidelity."

EVALUATING THE AUTHOR'S ARGUMENTS:

Ernest W. Lefever maintains that encouraging abstinence is the best way to slow the spread of AIDS. He cites the example of Uganda, which had a decrease in HIV infections after an abstinence program was started there in the late 1980s. He also points out, however, that Uganda's success in curbing AIDS appears to be slowing down. What has caused this slowing down, in Lefever's opinion? Do you agree with him? Or do you think there may be other reasons for an increase in HIV infections in Uganda? Explain your answer.

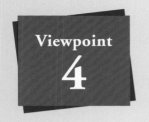

Abstinence-Only Programs Do Not Slow the Spread of AIDS

"Abstinence-only does not work. Abstinence-plus probably does."

The Economist

Teaching that abstinence is the sole way to prevent HIV infection will not stop the spread of AIDS, *The Economist* asserts in the following viewpoint. A series of recent studies reveals that pregnancies and sexually transmitted diseases (STDs) are widespread in students enrolled in abstinence-only education. "Abstinence-plus" programs, which encourage chastity but also include information on condoms and STD-prevention, are more effective at reducing risky behavior, the author maintains. *The Economist* is a weekly news and international affairs publication.

AS YOU READ, CONSIDER THE FOLLOWING QUESTIONS:

1. Why do some critics oppose "abstinence-plus" education, in the opinion of *The Economist*?
2. According to Dr. Kristen Underhill, cited by the authors, how do students enrolled in abstinence-only education compare with students who are not enrolled in sex-education programs in terms of pregnancies and STDs?
3. What drugs are researchers currently testing as possible HIV-preventative medicines, according to *The Economist*?

There can be no surer way of averting a sexually transmitted infection such as AIDS than avoiding sex. That much is obvious. And it is also convenient for religious lobbyists who believe that premarital sex is a sin. But is it realistic? Those lobbyists argue that a popular alternative—known in the jargon as "abstinence-plus"—which recommends chastity but also explains how to use condoms, is likely to make things worse by encouraging earlier intercourse. "Abstinence-only" teaching, they reckon, should be more effective.

That, of course, is a possibility. But it is a testable possibility. And Kristen Underhill and her colleagues at the University of Oxford have, over the past few months, been testing it. Their conclusion is that it is wrong. Abstinence-only does not work. Abstinence-plus probably does.

> **FAST FACT**
>
> Columbia University researchers report that virginity-pledge programs increase pledge-takers' risk for sexually transmitted diseases.

Studies on Abstinence Education

Last month [August 2007] Dr Underhill published a review of 13 trials involving 16,000 young people in America. The trials compared the sexual behaviour of those given an abstinence-only education with that of those who were provided with no information at all or with whatever their schools normally taught. Pregnancies were as numerous in both groups. Sexually transmitted diseases were as widespread. The number of sexual partners was equally high and unprotected sex just as common.

Having thus discredited abstinence-only teaching, Dr Underhill and her colleagues decided to evaluate the slightly more complicated message of "abstinence-plus" using 39 trials that involved 38,000-odd young people from the United States, Canada and the Bahamas. Their results are published in the current [September 2007] issue of [the] Public Library of Science Medicine [journal] PLoS Medicine.

Knowledge Decreases Risk

This tuition [instruction]—compared, as before, with whatever biology classes and playgrounds provide—reduced the number of pregnancies in three out of seven trials (the remaining four recorded no difference). Four out of 13 trials found that abstinence-plus-educated teenagers had fewer sexual partners, while the remainder showed no change. Fourteen studies reported that it increased condom use; 12 others reported no difference. Furthermore, in the vast majority of cases, abstinence-plus participants knew more about AIDS and HIV (the virus that causes the disease) than their peers did. And the tuition often reduced the frequency of anal sex (which brings a greater chance of passing on HIV than the vaginal option). In contrast to the fears of the protagonists of abstinence-only education, not one of the trials found that teenagers behaved in a riskier fashion in either the long or the short term after receiving abstinence-plus instruction.

Unfortunately (and surprisingly) only two of the studies addressed the question of disease transmission directly, and the numbers involved were too small to find a statistically significant difference between groups. Nevertheless, Dr Underhill's pair of reviews should make informative reading for policymakers. . . .

Teens of the Pure Love Alliance march in support of abstinence programs. Several research trials found that teens exposed to abstinence-plus programs had fewer sexual partners than those schooled in abstinence-only teaching.

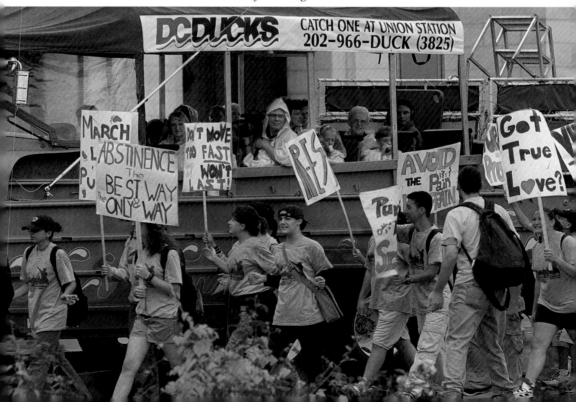

Abstinence Only Versus Comprehensive Sex Education

Abstinence-Plus Education

Abstinence-plus education programs explore the context for and meanings involved in sex.

* promote abstinence from sex
* acknowledge that many teenagers will become sexually active
* teach about contraception and condom use
* include discussions about contraception, abortion, sexually transmitted diseases and HIV

Abstinence-Only Education

Abstinence-only education programs include discussions of values, character building, and, in some cases, refusal skills.

* promote abstinence from sex
* do not acknowledge that many teenagers will become sexually active
* do not teach about contraception or condom use
* avoid discussions of abortion
* cite sexually transmitted diseases and HIV as reasons to remain abstinent

Taken from: Chris Collins et al. (Progressive Health Partners) and Stephen F. Morin (AIDS Research Institute, University of California–San Francisco), *Abstinence-Only vs. Comprehensive Sex Education: What Are the Arguments? What Is the Evidence?* Policy Monograph Series, March 2002.

A Dose of Prevention

Teaching people about what they might wear during intercourse is an important way of reducing the chance of them catching HIV. But teaching them, in addition, about what drugs they could take to reduce that risk may be added to the syllabus in the future. A vaccine is still a long way off, but four clinical trials—in Peru and Ecuador, Thailand, Botswana and also America—are assessing how well daily anti-retroviral pills, which are normally prescribed to control established HIV infections, prevent the virus infecting healthy people who do dangerous things. The results of these trials will be plugged into epidemiological computer models to assess the likely effect of various drug-distribution policies.

One model intended to do exactly that has already been built, by Ume Abbas and John Mellors of the University of Pittsburgh. It is designed to mimic a mature HIV epidemic in sub-Saharan Africa—which it did rather well when the researchers tested its output against data from Zambia, a country in which the epidemic has remained stable for a decade.

Writing in *PLoS Medicine*'s sister journal, *PLoS ONE*, Dr Abbas and Dr Mellors describe what happened when they added prophylactic [preventative] anti-retroviral drugs to the model. They experimented with different measures of drug efficacy and with different groups of people taking the pills.

Assuming that anti-retrovirals work 90% of the time and are taken by three-quarters of sexually active people, their model suggests that new HIV infections in sub-Saharan Africa would be cut by 74% over 10 years. Unfortunately, the idea of providing and delivering so many drugs to so many people is logistically implausible. And even if it could be done, it would cost about $6,000 per HIV infection averted—a lot of money in Africa.

However, giving the drug to the 16% of Africans who behave most riskily would be easier and could lead to a 29% reduction over a decade at only a tenth of that cost. A harsh calculation, but a realistic one—unlike expecting teenagers to give up sex because you tell them to.

EVALUATING THE AUTHORS' ARGUMENTS:

In this viewpoint *The Economist* argues that "abstinence-only" teaching will not slow the spread of HIV—yet also admits that promoting abstinence is a good strategy for preventing the spread of HIV. What points of agreement would this author share with Ernest W. Lefever, author of the previous selection? On what points would they disagree?

A Vaccine Can Help Slow the Spread of AIDS

Anthony S. Fauci, Margaret I. Johnston, and Gary J. Nabel

"Vaccines historically have been the most effective means to prevent and even eradicate infectious diseases."

In the following selection three medical researchers, Anthony S. Fauci, Margaret I. Johnston, and Gary J. Nabel, announce that a safe and effective HIV vaccine is on the horizon. Clinical trials indicate modest success with an experimental HIV vaccine, the authors report, and further research is likely to improve on these results. The recent discovery of new antibodies that can disable the AIDS virus might be the key to boosting the immune system's response to HIV infection. Fauci is director of the National Institute of Allergy and Infectious Diseases (NIAID) in Bethesda, Maryland. Johnston is director of the Vaccine Research Program in the Division of AIDS at NIAID. Nabel is director of the Dale and Betty Bumpers Vaccine Research Center at NIAID.

1. According to the authors, the experimental AIDS vaccine prevents HIV infection in what percentage of cases?
2. How do the newly discovered AIDS antibodies disable HIV, according to researchers?
3. What other HIV prevention tools are needed in addition to an effective AIDS vaccine, in the authors' opinion?

More people today have access to life-saving antiretroviral therapy for HIV/AIDS than ever before. Yet for every person who begins treatment for HIV infection, two to three others become newly infected. Treatment alone will not curtail the HIV/AIDS pandemic. To control and ultimately end this pandemic, we need a powerful array of proven HIV prevention tools that are widely accessible to all who would benefit from them.

Vaccines historically have been the most effective means to prevent and even eradicate infectious diseases. They safely and cost-effectively prevent illness, disability and death. We at the National Institute of Allergy and Infectious Diseases (NIAID), part of the National Institutes of Health, have been working for more than two decades with our colleagues worldwide to develop an HIV vaccine, and this research continues to rank among our top priorities.

FAST FACT

In lab tests, recently discovered antibodies have prevented 90 percent of circulating HIV strains from infecting human cells.

National HIV Vaccine Awareness Day [May 18, 2010] marks an opportunity to reflect on our progress, renew our commitment to finding an HIV vaccine, and personally thank the scientists, community educators, health care workers, and especially the many study volunteers who have dedicated their time and energy to this important endeavor. Only with the continued commitment of volunteers may we more effectively confront the global scourge of HIV/AIDS and pursue the goal of an HIV vaccine.

Progress in Research

We have witnessed significant progress in HIV vaccine research during the past year [2009–2010]. Notably, a major clinical trial in Thailand gave us the first indication that an experimental vaccine can protect some humans against HIV infection. With the participation of more than 16,000 volunteers, investigators found the vaccine to be 31 percent effective at preventing HIV infection. Although this level of protection is modest, it gives us hope that a safe and effective HIV vaccine is possible. The priority now is to try to understand how the vaccine induced protection against HIV infection in some individuals, and to build on those results.

The Thai trial demonstrated the power of large-scale clinical trials to advance HIV vaccine development and to answer fundamental scientific questions. Such trials are possible only through strategic partnerships among federal collaborators, nongovernmental organizations and the private sector. NIAID continues to pursue focused clinical HIV vaccine research through such partnerships.

A major clinical trial for an AIDS vaccine in Thailand in 2009–2010 has shown that the vaccine can protect some people against HIV infection.

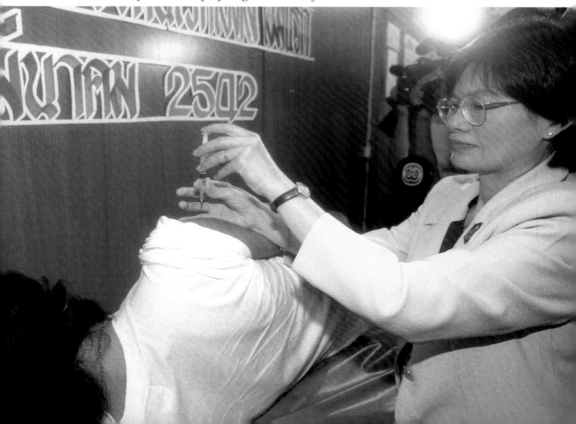

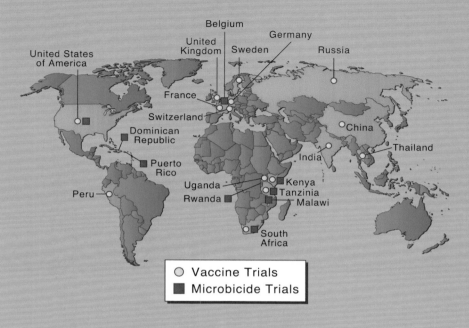

HIV Vaccine and Microbicide Trials Around the Globe

Belgium
Germany
United
Kingdom   Sweden   Russia
United States
of America
France
China
Switzerland
Thailand
Dominican
Republic   India
Puerto
Rico
Uganda   Kenya
Peru   Rwanda   Tanzinia
Malawi
South
Africa

○ Vaccine Trials
■ Microbicide Trials

Taken from: Global Advocacy for HIV Prevention, 2010. www.avac.org/ht/d/sp/i/189/pid/189.

New Antibodies

At the same time, we are bolstering our commitment to the basic laboratory research that provides a foundation for future vaccine development. In the past year, scientists at NIAID and elsewhere discovered several new antibodies able to neutralize diverse HIV strains that circulate worldwide.

These antibodies disable HIV by latching onto vulnerable sites on the virus. Some of these sites previously were unknown, so their discovery widens the field of targets that a vaccine could exploit. Current and future studies will determine whether scientists can develop HIV vaccines based on protein replicas of these targets, and whether the immune response to these vaccines might protect people from HIV infection. Many other studies also are under way to explore basic questions about HIV and its interaction with the immune system.

An Array of Methods Are Needed

As we recognize recent progress in HIV vaccine research and hope for continued advances, we must remember that a vaccine alone will not end the HIV/AIDS pandemic. If an HIV vaccine is developed, it will need to be used in concert with multiple other scientifically proven HIV prevention tools. NIAID continues to support research into an array of investigational HIV prevention methods, including pre-exposure prophylaxis [preventative treatment] with antiretroviral drugs, microbicides, and expanded HIV testing and treatment with linkage to care.

> **EVALUATING THE AUTHORS' ARGUMENTS:**
>
> The authors of this viewpoint, Anthony S. Fauci, Margaret I. Johnston, and Gary J. Nabel, are highly regarded scientific researchers. They feel optimistic about the future of an AIDS vaccine, even though the experimental vaccine they discuss is only 30 percent effective. In your opinion, do the credentials of these authors influence a reader's assessment of their argument? Explain.

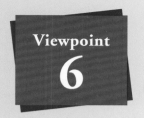

Viewpoint
6

An AIDS Vaccine Could Be Ineffective

Thomas H. Maugh II

"The new analysis, which was part of the trial protocol, showed that [the vaccine] seemed to reduce infections by only 26 percent [rather than by 31 percent]."

In the following viewpoint Thomas H. Maugh II discusses additional research results published after the initial announcement of the Thai AIDS vaccine trial results in September 2009. The percentage of effectiveness may now be lower than originally determined because, unlike the earlier analysis, Maugh reports, none of the original participants were excluded in the later analysis. The lower percentage of effectiveness may mean the results are not statistically significant and might have happened by chance. Maugh is a science and medical writer with *The Los Angeles Times.*

AS YOU READ, CONSIDER THE FOLLOWING QUESTIONS:
1. What does Dr. Raphael Dolin say about the overall findings of the Thai AIDS vaccine trial?
2. What does Dr. Otto Yang say about the Thai vaccine as a result of the new findings?
3. What were the components of the Thai AIDS vaccine, and how were they expected to perform?

A secondary analysis of data from the Thai AIDS vaccine trial—announced last month [September 2009] to much acclaim—suggests that the vaccine might provide some protection against the virus, but that the results are not statistically significant. In short, they could have resulted merely from chance.

Initial results from the trial involving more than 16,000 people had shown that the vaccine reduced infections by about 31 percent and that the results, though limited, were statistically significant. The new analysis, which was part of the trial protocol, showed that it seemed to reduce infections by only 26 percent.

Full results of the trial were published online in the *New England Journal of Medicine* and announced Tuesday at an AIDS vaccine conference in Paris.

A second analysis of the Thai AIDS vaccine trial has revealed that the treatment is not as promising as originally hoped.

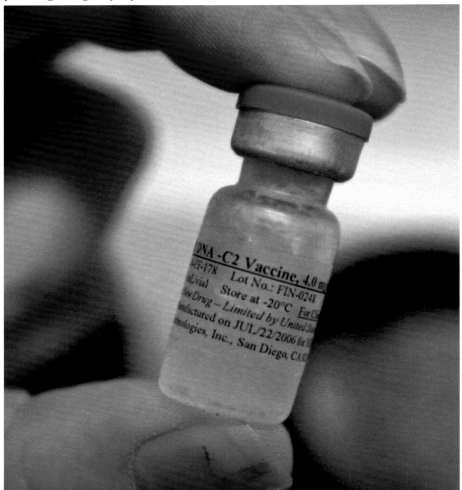

In an editorial accompanying the journal paper, Dr. Raphael Dolin of the Beth Israel Deaconess Medical Center in Boston said the overall findings are nonetheless "of potentially great importance to the field of HIV research" because they may yield information about the kinds of immune responses necessary to provide protection against the virus.

Dr. Otto Yang, an immunologist at the University of California at Los Angeles' Geffen School of Medicine, cautioned that "the results are weak enough that we need to be very careful about assigning too much optimism to them. . . . It seems not so likely that the vaccine really did what it was intended to do."

The trial, sponsored largely by the National Institute of Allergy and Infectious Diseases, combined two vaccines—each of which had individually proved ineffective in previous trials—in the hope that one would prime the immune system and the second would boost immunity.

The key difference between the two types of analyses is that the original one excluded seven patients who were found to have HIV infections at the time the study began. The new analysis, included all patients who were originally enrolled in the trial, producing the weaker results. Vaccine trials are typically analyzed both ways, and researchers expect to see statistically significant results from each analysis.

The fact that they did not in this case suggests that any effects of the vaccine were exceptionally modest.

EVALUATING THE AUTHORS' ARGUMENTS:

Compare this viewpoint by Thomas H. Maugh II with the preceding selection by Anthony S. Fauci, Margaret I. Johnson, and Gary J. Nabel, which deals with the same Thai AIDs vaccine trial. Should the Thai trial offer any hope to AIDS researchers and patients? Explain your answer using evidence from each viewpoint.

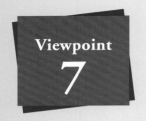

Stem Cell Therapy Could Slow the Spread of AIDS

Investor's Business Daily

"A patient who was treated with adult stem cells appears to now be free of the HIV virus."

The national US newspaper *Investor's Business Daily* reports here on a patient HIV-positive for ten years and undergoing antiviral treatments who, in 2007, received transplanted adult stem cells from a specifically-selected donor. The donor has a gene mutation that confers immunity to HIV. As of early 2009, the patient remains HIV-free and requires no antiviral medications. Stem-cell transplants are too risky for most AIDS patients, the authors note, but ongoing research with adult stem cells may lead to gene therapies that result in controlling HIV.

AS YOU READ, CONSIDER THE FOLLOWING QUESTIONS:
1. According to the authors, why did the HIV-positive patient who received the experimental stem-cell transplant need to stop taking antiviral drugs?
2. What was unique about the stem cells that were used in this experimental transplant, according to *Investor's Business Daily*?
3. In the opinion of Dr. Gero Hutter, quoted in this article, how was the HIV-positive patient faring two years after the stem-cell transplant?

A patient who was treated with adult stem cells appears to now be free of the HIV virus and the need for a lifetime of drugs. And there was no need for the destruction of human embryos.

Up to now, AIDS was a disease that could be controlled only with drugs. There were no cures, and the best that could be hoped for was for a controlled remission. A report published Wednesday [in February 2009] in the *New England Journal of Medicine* offers new hope in the treatment of that deadly disease.

Bone Marrow Stem Cells

The 42-year-old HIV patient described in the report was treated with antiviral drugs for 10 years since being diagnosed. In July 2006, he developed leukemia and was given chemotherapy. That controlled his leukemia, but led to kidney and liver failure. When doctors halted the antiviral drugs, his HIV levels spiked again.

Bone marrow stem cells in just 1 percent of people contain a gene mutation that makes a transplant recipient immune to the HIV virus.

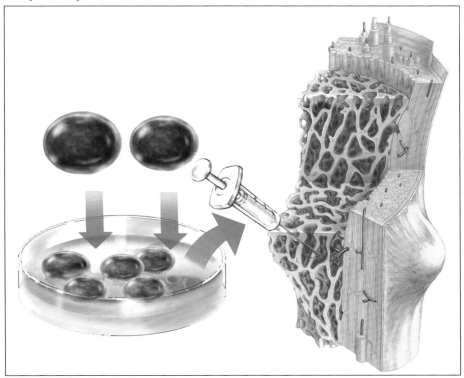

When they resumed his antiviral drugs, the leukemia returned, so doctors decided to try a stem cell transplant using bone marrow. Adult stem cells from bone marrow have the ability to form blood cells, including the white blood cells that fight infection. These are the cells the HIV virus attacks, crippling patients' immune systems.

The difference between this and other adult stem cell transplants is that this time, doctors deliberately sought out a donor who had a naturally occurring gene mutation that confers natural immunity to the HIV virus.

The mutation cripples a receptor known as CCR5 that is found on the surface of cells attacked by HIV and helps the virus enter the cell. The mutation occurs in 1% to 3% of white people of European descent. It worked beyond expectations.

New Ways of Controlling Illness

"The patient is fine," said Dr. Gero Hutter of Charite Universitatsmedizin Berlin [a university hospital in Germany]. "Today, two years after his transplantation, he is still without any signs of HIV disease and without anti-retroviral medication."

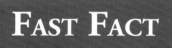

FAST FACT

Delta 32 is a genetic mutation in which white blood cells lack the surface receptors that allow HIV to invade the immune system.

While Hutter admits the stem cell transplant procedure is too risky to try in most AIDS patients, some are so sick it's worth the risk. This experiment has pointed researchers to a new way of controlling HIV such as gene therapy to modify cells so they lack the CCR5 receptor.

This discovery follows on the heels of another study published last month [January 2009] in the British medical journal *Lancet* detailing how adult stem cells transplanted into early-phase multiple sclerosis [MS] patients stabilized, and in some cases reversed, the debilitating neurological disorder.

In clinical trials, a team of scientists led by Richard Burt of Northwestern University in Chicago essentially rebuilt the immune systems of 21 adults who had failed to respond to standard drug treatments. They all had MS for at least five years.

Some Diseases and Conditions Successfully Treated Using Adult Stem Cells

Diseases and Conditions
• Brain cancer
• Breast cancer
• Lymphoma
• Leukemia
• Multiple sclerosis
• Systemic lupus
• Crohn's disease
• Parkinson's disease
• Sickle-cell anemia
• Spinal-cord injuries
• Limb gangrene
• Stroke damage
• Heart damage

Taken from: Marie Godfrey, Gene Forum, www.geneforum.org/node/135.

The treatments removed defective white blood cells that, rather than protecting the body, were attacking the fatty sheath, called myelin, that protects the nervous system. The immune systems were then replenished with haemopoietic stem cells [those involved in the formation of blood cells] extracted from the patients' bone marrow. These cells are capable of giving rise to any form of mature blood cell.

After an average follow-up period of three years, 17 of the 21 patients improved by at least one point on a standard disability scale. None got worse. The procedure "not only seems to prevent neurological progression, but also appears to reverse neurological disability," the study concluded.

Important Research

These advances show once again that embryonic stem cell research [ESCR] is not necessarily the most promising avenue of research or the only one that should be pursued. This and other discoveries come without the moral baggage that ESCR carries with it and without the federal funds that supporters say are indispensable.

Research over more than two decades has failed to produce any medically valuable treatments or therapies. Applications of adult stem cells, by contrast, have been useful in hundreds of actual therapies and treatments of real people suffering from a variety of ailments. Yet adult stem cell successes are ignored. Hopefully that will change.

EVALUATING THE AUTHOR'S ARGUMENTS:

According to Dr. Gero Hutter, cited in this selection, stem-cell transplants are too dangerous to use in most AIDS patients. Does this fact undercut the author's main assertion that stem-cell therapy can benefit people infected with HIV? Why or why not?

Chapter 3

How Should the Global AIDS Epidemic Be Addressed?

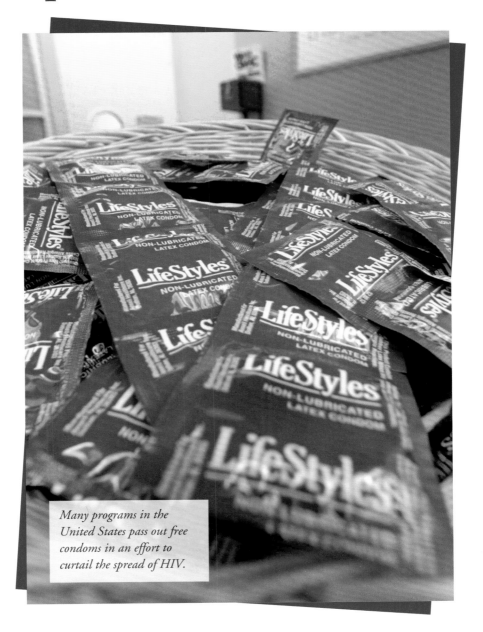

Many programs in the United States pass out free condoms in an effort to curtail the spread of HIV.

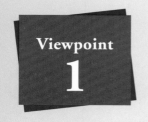

Condom Use Should Be Encouraged

USA Today

"An effective campaign to curb the HIV epidemic cannot function without condoms."

Curbing the global AIDS epidemic will require effective education programs about HIV prevention, *USA Today* reports in the following viewpoint. Encouraging the use of condoms is a necessary part of such a plan, the author asserts, as the condom is the only available technology that protects against HIV. Raising awareness and promoting condom use among at-risk populations should also be a key goal because it will help to reduce the number of new infections. *USA Today* is a monthly magazine of news, culture, and political opinion.

AS YOU READ, CONSIDER THE FOLLOWING QUESTIONS:

1. According to Lester Brown, cited by the author, what should be the first goal in stemming the AIDS epidemic?
2. In developing nations, which groups are most likely to become infected with and to spread HIV, according to the author?
3. What other policies would help to curb the global AIDS epidemic, in the author's view?

USA Today, "Curbing the HIV Scourge: Ignorance and Wrongheaded Policies Continue to Endanger Millions," *USA Today (Magazine),* vol. 137, no. 2765, February 2009, p. 16. Copyright © 2009 by Society for the Advancement of Education. Reproduced by permission.

The key to curbing the AIDS epidemic, which has so disrupted economic and social progress in Africa, is education about prevention, contends Lester R. Brown, president of [environmental organization] Earth Policy Institute, Washington, D.C., and author of *Plan B: Rescuing a Planet Under Stress and a Civilization in Trouble*. How the disease is transmitted is well-known; it is not a medical mystery. In Africa, where there once was a stigma associated with even mentioning AIDS, governments are beginning to design effective prevention education programs. The first goal is to reduce the number of new infections quickly, dropping it below the number of deaths, thus shrinking the number of those who are capable of infecting others.

Targeting At-Risk Populations

Concentrating on the groups in a society who are most likely to spread the disease is particularly effective, Brown suggests. In Africa, infected truck drivers who travel far from home for extended periods often engage in commercial sex, spreading the HIV virus that causes

Free condoms are distributed to people in Lagos, Nigeria. This African country's people are considered to be particularly at risk of contracting HIV because 5 percent of the population is already infected.

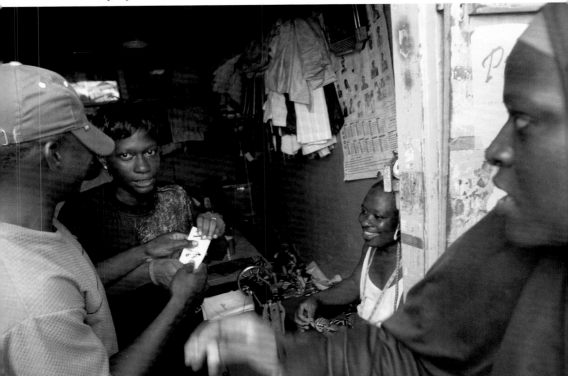

AIDS from one country to another—making them a primary target group for reducing infections. Sex workers obviously are involved in the spread of the disease as well. In India, for instance, the country's 2,000,000 female prostitutes have an average of two encounters per day, making them a key group to educate about HIV risks and the life-saving value of using a condom. Another target group is the military, adds Brown. After soldiers become infected, usually from engaging in commercial sex, they return to their home communities and spread the virus further. In Nigeria, where the adult HIV infection rate is five percent, former Pres. Olusegun Obasanjo required free distribution of condoms to all military personnel. A fourth target group, intravenous drug users who share needles, figures prominently in the spread of the virus in the former Soviet republics.

A Small Price to Pay

At the most fundamental level, dealing with the HIV threat requires roughly 10,000,000,000 condoms a year in the developing world and Eastern Europe. Including those needed for contraception adds another 2,000,000,000, but only 2,500,000,000 condoms are being distributed.

Since they cost just three cents each, a mere $285,000,000 could take care of the shortfall. In one study, Population Action International [an international organization that advocates for access to reproductive health care] notes that "the costs of getting condoms into the hands of users—which involves improving access, logistics and distribution capacity, raising awareness, and promoting use—is many times that of the supplies themselves." If we assume that these costs are six times the price of the condoms, filling this gap still would be only $2,000,000,000, a small price to pay considering how many lives could be spared, Brown insists.

Yet, even though condoms are the only technology available to prevent the spread of HIV, the U.S. government under the [George

W.] Bush Administration deemphasized their use, insisting that abstinence be given top priority, Brown laments. While encouraging abstinence is important, an effective campaign to curb the HIV epidemic cannot function without condoms.

A Few Successes

Meanwhile, one of the few African countries to lower the HIV infection rate successfully after the epidemic became well established is Uganda. Under the leadership of Pres. Yoweri Museveni, the share of adults infected has dropped from a peak of 13% in the early 1990s to around four percent today [February 2009]. Zambia also appears to be making progress in reducing infection rates among young people as a result of a concerted national campaign led by church groups. Senegal, which acted early and decisively to check the spread of the virus, has an infection rate among adults of less than one percent today. It is a model for other African countries.

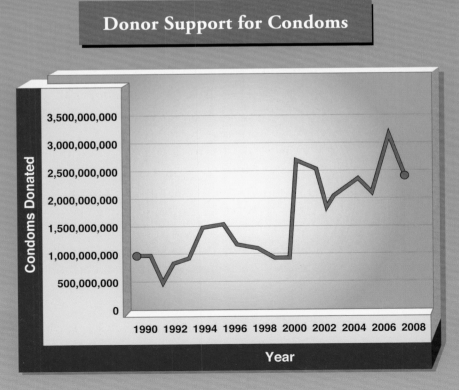

Taken from: Avert.org, "Condoms: Effectiveness, History, and Availability," July 14, 2010.

The financial resources and medical personnel currently available to treat people who already are HIV-positive are limited compared with the need. For example, of the 4,700,000 people who exhibited symptoms of AIDS in sub-Saharan Africa, only 500,000 were receiving the antiretroviral drug treatment that widely is available in industrial countries. However, this was up threefold from just 12 months earlier. The increase is part of a worldwide effort by the World Health Organization to reach out to millions of AIDS victims, Brown points out.

There is a growing body of evidence that the prospect of treatment encourages people to get tested for HIV. It also raises awareness and understanding of the disease and how it is transmitted. If people know they are infected, they may try to avoid infecting others. To the extent that treatment extends life—about 15 years in the U.S., for instance—it not only is the humanitarian thing to do, it makes economic sense. Once society has invested in the rearing, education, and on-the-job training of an individual, the value of extending the working lifetime is high.

Africa is paying a heavy price for its delayed response to the epidemic. It is a window on the future of other countries—such as India and China—if they do not move quickly to contain the virus that already is well established within their borders, cautions Brown.

EVALUATING THE AUTHORS' ARGUMENTS:

The author argues that education and outreach to the groups that are most likely to spread HIV is an especially effective way to curb the global AIDS pandemic. In light of what you have read elsewhere in this text, do you agree? Or do you think that there are other strategies that would have a greater impact? Explain.

Condom Use Should Not Be Encouraged

M.J. Ferrari

"Numerous reports . . . have proven the ineffectiveness of condoms in stemming the tide of AIDS."

M.J. Ferrari, the author of the following selection, maintains that condoms are ineffective against the spread of AIDS. In Africa the most successful campaigns against HIV have emphasized chastity and teaching that sex is not a recreational activity, notes Ferrari. In Ferrari's opinion, promoting the use of condoms is actually dangerous because they create a false sense of security and do not reliably protect against sexually transmitted diseases. Ferrari is a canon (church-law) lawyer and medical doctor who frequently contributes to *Catholic Insight* magazine.

AS YOU READ, CONSIDER THE FOLLOWING QUESTIONS:

1. How does the Youth Alive program of Malawi teach African youth to avoid HIV, according to the author?
2. Why does Ferrari disapprove of Bishop Kevin Dowling of the Catholic diocese of Rustenberg, South Africa?
3. According to a Joint United Nations Programme on HIV/AIDS (UNAIDS) study cited in this article, what percentage of the time are condoms ineffective against HIV?

M.J. Ferrari, "Southern Africa and AIDS: Why Chastity, Not Condoms, Is the Answer," *Catholic Insight*, vol. 15, no. 9, October 2007, pp. 19–20. Copyright © 2007 by *Catholic Insight*. Reproduced by permission.

A IDS is endemic in Africa and the Missionaries of the Immaculate Conception (MIC), with headquarters in Montreal, and the Children's Fund of Canada (JMJ) are trying to do something about it. On March 6, 2007, during a side event at the 51st meeting of the Commission on the Status of Women in New York, JMJ Children's Fund of Canada, Inc. presented a workshop showing how young people in Malawi are learning to change their lives and avoid AIDS.

FAST FACT

Condoms are not 100 percent effective and therefore cannot provide absolute protection against any sexually transmitted disease.

Known as "Youth Alive," the program consists of four days of intensive and interactive workshops for young people, teaching them how to change their lifestyles. For African youth, this involves overcoming cultural practices that are harmful and deeply ingrained. It also teaches them to ignore large billboards, seen in most towns and villages in Malawi, promoting sex with condoms. They are learning that sex is not a recreational activity.

Programs That Work

The program has achieved major successes. The best known is in Uganda where, in 1986, President Yoweri Museveni embarked on a nationwide tour to tell people it was their patriotic duty to avoid AIDS. He instructed them to avoid sex before marriage, be faithful to their spouses and to use condoms if necessary. The health minister focused on providing safe blood products and educating people about the risks of indiscriminate sex. In 1991, the prevalence of AIDS among pregnant women was 21 per cent, while the national average was 15 per cent.

In 1992, the Ugandan government adopted a multisectoral approach, enlisting the support of influential people in the media and the arts to promote the program. Various government departments (agriculture, internal affairs, justice, etc.) established individual AIDS-control program units. In 1997, a special study using anti-retroviral drugs to prevent mother-child transmission of HIV was instituted. Over the next several years, the incidence of AIDS in

Uganda decreased by 80 per cent. Unable or unwilling to accept the implications of the program, some people in America are trying to discredit these statistics. They are not reliable, they say. Are statistics anywhere in Africa reliable? If statistics were acceptable before this major advance, why are they not acceptable now?

In any case, Youth Alive Zambia credits Youth Alive Uganda for the program. In 2000, Sister Yvonne Ayotte, MIC, sent 10 young people to Zambia to learn about Youth Alive. To quote from the little booklet prepared by the young people last year: "With time, Youth Alive Mzuzu began to reach out to other youths in various parts of Malawi with their Behaviour Change Program (BCP). It also started training youths from other parts of the country, at the invitation of the bishops, to train others" and is now a national organization.

Effects on Youth

To assist them in their choices, during the four-day workshops the young people review what their lives have been like. When asked to illustrate this, one young person drew a graveyard with crosses. They

A teacher writes "AIDS Kills" on a blackboard at a Youth Alive workshop that teaches students in Malawi, Africa, how to make lifestyle changes that reduce the chance of contracting an HIV infection.

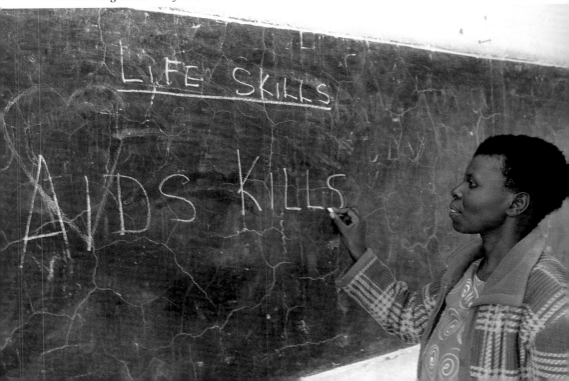

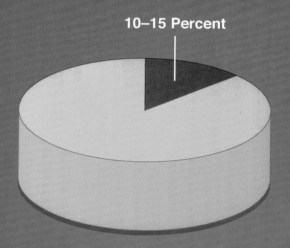

HIV Transmission Rate in Condom-Using Couples Where One Partner Is HIV Positive

10–15 Percent

Taken from: Go Ask Alice, Columbia University's Health Q&A Internet Service, 2002. www.goaskalice.columbia.edu.2002.

also look at how life is now and what it could be. They are taught that sex is not a recreational activity and that they should look for alternatives. Youth Alive clubs have been formed in secondary schools, featuring football, netball, debates and quizzes. . . .

The JMJ workshop in New York was well attended and the question period was lively. One woman asked: "What can a woman do, whose husband has AIDS? Do you recommend the use of condoms?"

Bishop Dowling

Bishop Kevin Dowling of the Catholic diocese of Rustenberg, South Africa, is distributing condoms to the poor women who tell him "the only way to eat is boyfriends."

"How can we recommend the use of condoms when they are not reliable, when even the New York State Department of Health tells young people in one of their pamphlets addressed to teenagers: "Abstinence is the only 100 per cent sure way not to catch . . . STD(s). . . . Using a condom every time can reduce the chances of passing HIV or other STD(s) . . . but you will (still) be at risk."

Promoting condoms merely creates a false sense of security, and nourishes the obsession created by the media that if one is not sexually active, he or she is emotionally or psychologically handicapped.

The woman from South Africa who asked the question is between a rock and a hard place, and is typical of the women facing Bishop Dowling. But the bishop is doing them no favours if he does not promote Church teaching. Ever since Peter's time, the Apostles and their followers have been instructed to take up their crosses, even in a hedonistic society. Instead of gluttony, the Church promotes fasting; in place of lust, chastity; in place of pride, humility; in place of self-indulgence, self-restraint—like Christ taking up his cross. Anything else is betrayal.

And when the woman finds she is HIV-positive, will she go back to Bishop Dowling and tell him: "I shall never trust you again"?

Condoms Are Not Reliable

Recent news headlines have reinforced the position that, even apart from the moral implications, a reliance on condoms is dangerous from a health standpoint. The South African health department recently recalled some twenty million potentially defective condoms that had been approved by an official accused of taking bribes from the manufacturer.

The situation was reported to have caused panic in neighbouring Zimbabwe when the condoms were found to have made their way there. "Many lives have been put at risk because of it," said the country's deputy minister of health and child welfare.

In Washington, D.C., more than 100,000 condoms given away in a citywide campaign have been sent back because of complaints the packaging was damaged and could have made the products ineffective.

These scandals follow numerous reports that have proven the ineffectiveness of condoms in stemming the tide of AIDS, sexually transmitted diseases and unplanned pregnancies:

- Researchers at the University of Washington found that infection rates for a new sexually transmitted disease, *Mycoplasma genitalium,* were four times higher among those who used condoms than among those who did not.

- A study published in the *New England Journal of Medicine* found that of every 100 women who use condoms 100 per cent of the time for one year, 37 were infected with human papilloma virus.
- Prize-winning medical journalist Sue Ellin Browder has concluded "there's no good evidence that condoms will reverse population-wide epidemics like those in sub-Saharan Africa." Instead, she said, the explosion in HIV/AIDS infection rates can be directly linked to reliance on condom use as a virus preventative.
- The first lady of Kenya, Lucy Kibaki, said, "This gadget called the condom . . . is causing the spread of AIDS in this country."
- Medical experts presenting their findings on the HIV pandemic three years ago [in 2004] found the availability of condoms statistically increases promiscuity and the risk of contracting the virus. Declines in incidence of HIV in Uganda, meanwhile, "are linked to behaviour change and include primary risk avoidance, with a 65 per cent decline in casual sex."
- A United Nations AIDS agency (UNAIDS) study found that condoms are ineffective against the spread of HIV an estimated 10 per cent of the time. The lead author said, "We should be talking about safer sex, not safe sex, with condoms."

EVALUATING THE AUTHOR'S ARGUMENTS:

M.J. Ferrari praises Youth Alive, a program of interactive workshops that teaches African youths how to overcome cultural practices that would put them at risk of becoming infected with HIV. One of the lessons teaches students to ignore billboards that promote the use of condoms. Do you think that this approach to AIDS prevention would work for the young people in the city where you reside? Why or why not?

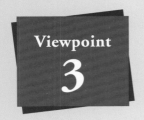

Individual Responsibility Should Be Encouraged

*"[AIDS]
can only be
overcome by
individuals
taking
responsibility
for their own
lives and
the lives of
those around
them."*

Jacob Zuma

The following viewpoint is excerpted from a 2009 public address by South African president Jacob Zuma as he announced a new program allowing universal access to HIV testing and treatment. Zuma asserts that prevention is the most powerful tool against the AIDS epidemic, and he implores all South Africans to take personal responsibility for protecting themselves, their loved ones, and their fellow citizens from HIV. All citizens should learn their HIV status, avoid risky behavior, and, if needed, undergo medical treatment, says Zuma. AIDS, he concludes, must be overcome "one individual at a time."

AS YOU READ, CONSIDER THE FOLLOWING QUESTIONS:

1. What has happened to the average life expectancy of South Africans since the beginning of the AIDS era, according to Zuma?
2. What does Zuma ask parents and heads of households to do in light of the AIDS epidemic?
3. Why does Zuma ask his audience to "remember to uphold the rights of women and children"?

Today [December 1, 2009] we join millions of people across the globe to mark World AIDS Day.

We join multitudes who have determined that this epidemic cannot be overcome without a concerted and coordinated effort.

We join millions who understand that the epidemic is not merely a health challenge. It is a challenge with profound social, cultural and economic consequences.

It is an epidemic that affects entire nations. Yet it touches on matters that are intensely personal and private.

Unlike many others, HIV and AIDS cannot be overcome simply by improving the quality of drinking water, or eradicating mosquitoes, or mass immunisation.

It can only be overcome by individuals taking responsibility for their own lives and the lives of those around them.

Fellow South Africans, as a country, we have done much to tackle HIV and AIDS.

In every sector of society, there are individuals and groups who have worked tirelessly to educate, advocate, care, treat, prevent and to break the stigma that still surrounds the epidemic. . . .

Working with other sectors through the South African National AIDS Council, we have managed to harness unity in confronting this scourge.

The amount of resources dedicated to prevention, treatment and care has increased with each successive year.

But it is not enough. Much more needs to be done.

We need extraordinary measures to reverse the trends we are seeing in the health profile of our people.

We know that the situation is serious. We have seen the statistics.

We know that the average life expectancy of South Africans has been falling, and that South Africans are dying at a young age.

We have seen the child-headed and granny-headed households, and have witnessed the pain and displacement of orphans and vulnerable children.

These facts are undeniable. We should not be tempted to downplay the statistics and impact or to deny the reality that we face.

At the same time, the epidemic is not about statistics. It is about people, about families, and communities.

It is about our loved ones.

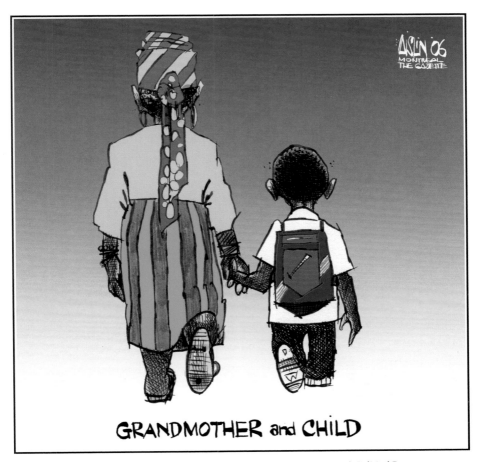

GRANDMOTHER and CHILD

"New African Family," cartoon by Aislin, *The Montreal Gazette,* August 15, 2006, PoliticalCartoons.com. Copyright © 2006 by Aislin and CagleCartoons.com. All rights reserved.

For many families, it is a burden that they have to bear alone, fearful of discrimination and stigma.

Dear Compatriots, now is not the time to lament. It is the time to act decisively, and to act together.

Our message is simple. We have to stop the spread of HIV. We must reduce the rate of new infections. Prevention is our most powerful weapon against the epidemic.

All South Africans should take steps to ensure that they do not become infected, that they do not infect others and that they know their status.

Each individual must take responsibility for protection against HIV. To the youth, the future belongs to you.

Be responsible and do not expose yourself to risks.

Parents and heads of households, let us be open with our children and educate them about HIV and how to prevent it.

Ladies and gentlemen, we are still marking the 16 days of activism against violence on women and children.[1] During this period, it is important that we also remember to uphold the rights of women and children, including their right to protection from infection with HIV.

Many women are unable to negotiate for protection due to unequal power relations in relationships.

As we mark the International Day of Persons with Disabilities on Thursday, the 3rd of December, let us remember the impact of HIV on persons with disability.

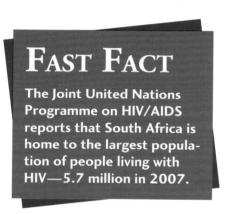

FAST FACT

The Joint United Nations Programme on HIV/AIDS reports that South Africa is home to the largest population of people living with HIV—5.7 million in 2007.

We have to tailor government programmes and messages to also speak to the needs of this sector.

Fellow South Africans, to take our response a step forward, we are launching a massive campaign to mobilise all South Africans to get tested for HIV.

Every South African should know his or her HIV status. . . .

In order to meet the need for testing and treatment, we will work to ensure that all the health institutions in the country are ready to receive and assist patients and not just a few accredited ARV [antiretroviral drug] centres. Any citizen should be able to move into any health centre and ask for counselling, testing and even treatment if needed. . . .

What does this all mean? It means that we will be treating significantly larger numbers of HIV positive patients. It means that people will live longer and more fulfilling lives.

What does it NOT mean? It does not mean that we should be irresponsible in our sexual practices.

1. The 16 Days of Activism international campaign, which runs annually from November 25th to December 10th, calls for an end to violence against women. South Africa also uses this campaign to focus on the problem of child abuse.

It does not mean that people do not have to practice safer sex. It does not mean that people should not use condoms consistently and correctly during every sexual encounter.

We can eliminate the scourge of HIV if all South Africans take responsibility for their actions.

I need to re-emphasise at this point that we must intensify our prevention efforts if we are to turn off the tap of new HIV and TB [tuberculosis] infections. Prevention is our most powerful and effective weapon.

We have to overcome HIV the same way that it spreads—one individual at a time. We have to really show that all of us are responsible.

The HIV tests are voluntary and they are confidential. We know that it is not easy. It is a difficult decision to take.

But it is a decision that must be taken by people from all walks of life, of all races, all social classes, all positions in society. HIV does not discriminate.

I am making arrangements for my own test. I have taken HIV tests before, and I know my status. I will do another test soon as

South African president Jacob Zuma, center, at a World AIDS Day event in Praetoria, South Africa. In 2009 Zuma announced universal access to HIV education, testing, and treatment for everyone in his country.

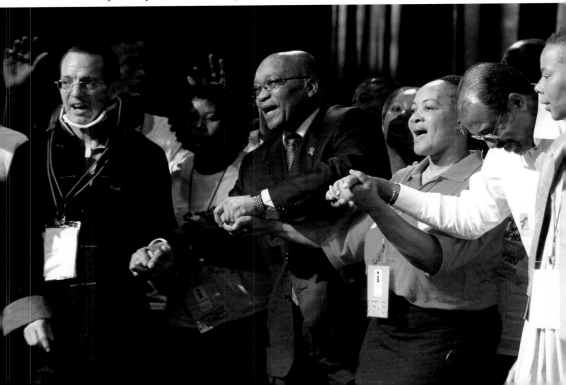

part of this new campaign. I urge you to start planning for your own tests. . . .

Fellow South Africans, another moment in our history, in another context, the liberation movement observed that the time comes in the life of any nation when there remain only two choices: submit or fight.

That time has now come in our struggle to overcome AIDS.

Let us declare now, as we declared then, that we shall not submit.

We have no choice but to deploy every effort, mobilise every resource, and utilise every skill that our nation possesses, to ensure that we prevail in this struggle for the health and prosperity of our nation.

History has demonstrated the strength of a nation united and determined.

We are a capable, innovative and motivated people.

Together we fought and defeated a system so corrupt and reviled that it was described as a crime against humanity.

Together we can overcome this challenge.

Let today be the dawn of a new era.

Let there be no more shame, no more blame, no more discrimination and no more stigma.

Let the politicisation and endless debates about HIV and AIDS stop.

Let this be the start of an era of openness, of taking personal responsibility, and of working together in unity to prevent HIV infections and to deal with its impact.

Working together, we can achieve these goals!

EVALUATING THE AUTHOR'S ARGUMENTS:

What effect does Jacob Zuma's use of repeated words and phrases have on you as a reader? Do the technique and tone of his speech make his argument more compelling? Why or why not?

More Funding Is Needed to Curtail AIDS

Charleston Gazette

"Today, [donors] are giving less."

The global fight against AIDS is in danger of falling apart due to cuts in funding, reports the *Charleston Gazette* in the following selection. Donating nations are giving less money than they were in the past, and some countries, such as the United States, are planning to cut contributions further. If this trend continues, most sub-Saharan African nations will be forced to cut back on the number of HIV victims that receive care. The United States and the international community must recommit to providing the financial backing that supports the struggle against AIDS, the *Gazette* concludes. The *Gazette* is a newspaper in Charleston, West Virginia.

AS YOU READ, CONSIDER THE FOLLOWING QUESTIONS:

1. According to the Joint United Nations Programme on HIV/ AIDS director Michel Sidibe, how much will it cost each year to control the spread of HIV?
2. According to the author, how many people in Uganda are in need of treatment for HIV? How many of them are receiving treatment?
3. How much is the Iraq War costing US taxpayers, according to economist Joseph Stiglitz?

Over the decade [2000–2009], glimmers of hope emerged that HIV/AIDS might be controlled and prevented from spreading. Today, those hopes might be disappearing.

Donors around the world were giving about $10 billion a year. Today, they are giving less.

The [Barack] Obama administration plans to cut $50 million from U.S. contributions to fight AIDS, according to the proposed 2011 budget.

> **FAST FACT**
>
> The Joint United Nations Programme on HIV/AIDS has found that cuts in funding often lead to stopping and restarting of HIV treatment, which can cause drug resistance and increased HIV transmission.

Michel Sidibe, executive director of UNAIDS [Joint United Nations Programme on HIV/AIDS], a United Nations program based in Geneva [Switzerland], believes it would take $27 billion a year to control the spreading epidemic, according to a May 9 [2010] article in *The New York Times.*

Hopes for a solution rose as drugs that once cost $12,000 a year to help an HIV victim dropped to less than $100.

Falling Apart?

Almost a decade ago, U.N. Secretary Kofi Annan formed the Global Fund and President George W. Bush created the President's Emergency Plan for AIDS Relief, called PEPFAR.

Today, though, the initiatives of Annan and Bush are disappearing.

"What I see is making me very scared," Sidibe said.

"Uganda is the first and most obvious example of how the war on global AIDS is falling part," the *Times* stated.

In Uganda, only 200,000 of 500,000 people who need treatment get it. And each year, another 110,000 Ugandans are infected with the deadly disease.

A lack of funds soon will force Kenya, Mozambique, Nigeria, Swaziland, Tanzania and Botswana to cut back on the number of victims they can help.

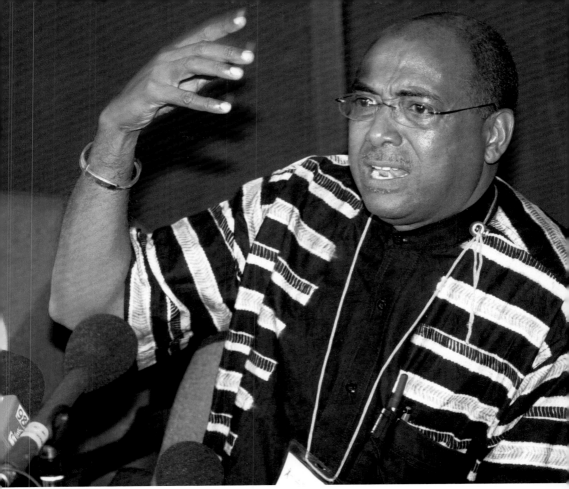

Executive director of UNAIDS Michel Sidibe addresses a press conference about AIDS. Sidibe believes it will take $27 billion a year to control the AIDS epidemic.

More Is Spent on War than on Controlling AIDS

The $27 billion that Sidibe estimates is needed to control AIDS is miniscule compared to trillions of dollars the U.S. government is spending to wage wars in Iraq and Afghanistan.

The Iraq war alone will cost taxpayers more than $3 trillion, according to Nobel Prize–winning economist Joseph Stiglitz.

Earlier this year [2010], the monthly costs of the U.S. war in Afghanistan began to exceed the monthly costs in Iraq.

A Critical Juncture

"The U.S. government commitment to PEPFAR has stagnated despite earlier promises of a $1 billion increase in desperately needed

In 71 surveyed countries, the 3.4 million people reported to be on treatment are but a minority of those who need it.

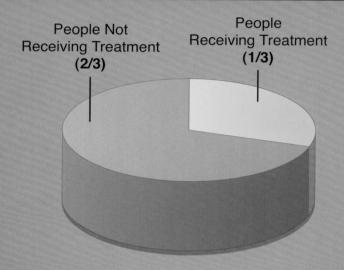

People Not
Receiving Treatment
(2/3)

People
Receiving Treatment
(1/3)

Taken from: UNAIDS and the World Bank, "The Global Economic Crisis and HIV Prevention and Treatment Programmes: Vulnerabilities and Impact," June 2009.

funds," according to a July 2009 report published by Doctors Without Borders, a charitable group.

"Three million people are on treatment today despite the fact that many had said it was impossible to treat in resource-poor settings. . . .

"At this critical juncture, the international community must reaffirm its commitment to providing treatment and care for people living with HIV/AIDS," the Doctors Without Borders report concludes.

Apart from any other reason, the U.S. government might generate a lot more good will around the world by spending more money to save the lives of AIDS victims than spending money to escalate wars.

This selection from the *Charleston Gazette* maintains that curtailing the AIDS pandemic will require more financial contributions from the United States and other affluent nations. In the preceding viewpoint Jacob Zuma emphasizes the importance of individual responsibility in fighting HIV. Who are the audiences for these respective viewpoints? Do you think that an awareness of audience affects how these authors approach their topics? Explain.

Access to AIDS Medicines Must Be Increased

Doctors Without Borders

"A sustained response to HIV/AIDS includes an obligation to put people on treatment and to continue treatment as medically required."

Doctors Without Borders/Médecins Sans Frontières (MSF) is an international medical humanitarian organization started by doctors and journalists in France in 1971. In the following selection MSF argues that all people must have access to effective HIV drugs if world leaders truly want to curb the AIDS epidemic. The medical crisis is ongoing because the majority of people who need HIV treatment are not receiving it, the authors point out. Global health guidelines now recommend that people receive antiretroviral drugs in earlier stages of the disease; furthermore, HIV patients may need stronger medicines and more frequent monitoring in the years to come. Providing this kind of treatment will require greater support from donors and from the international community, the authors conclude.

Ten years ago [in 2000], on the heels of Médecins Sans Frontières (MSF) being awarded the Nobel Peace Prize—and largely in response to the inequalities surrounding access to AIDS treatment between rich and poor countries—MSF launched the Campaign for Access to Essential Medicines. Its sole purpose has been to push for access to, and the development of life-saving and life-prolonging medicines, diagnostics and vaccines for patients in MSF programmes and beyond.

HIV/AIDS is a lifelong disease, and although there is no cure, treatment with antiretroviral drugs (ARVs) prolongs and improves the quality of life.

AIDS treatment in developing countries began roughly a decade ago, normally as small pilot projects and in the face of widespread scepticism about its feasibility in resource-poor settings. MSF was one of the first organisations to provide antiretroviral therapy (ART) in developing countries, starting with projects in Thailand and South Africa in 2000.

A Persistent Emergency

MSF now provides treatment to 140,000 people in more than 30 countries and today a total of four million people across the developing world are on ART. While this represents important progress, an approximately further six million people in immediate need of treatment are a testament to the persistent emergency. With growing numbers of patients in developing countries having been on treatment for five years or longer, new challenges are emerging to ensure their long-term survival. In India alone nearly 240,000 people are accessing first-line ART under the national AIDS treatment programme.

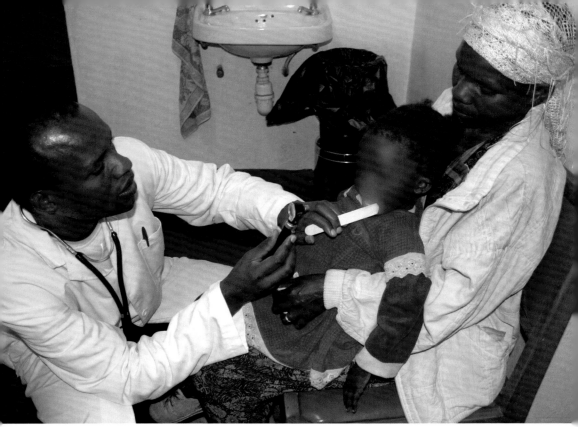

An HIV-positive child is examined at a clinic in Kenya, Africa, run by Médecins Sans Frontières (MSF). The organization's sole mission is to promote the development of life-saving diagnostics and treatments for patients in MSF programs.

Delivering ART to millions of people in developing countries was made possible because treatment was brought close to where people lived, drug costs came down dramatically, and treatment was simplified; several medicines were combined into one pill (a fixed-dose combination, or FDC). And in order to address the shortages of medical staff in many countries, tasks are being shifted in many places, so that nurses or nurse aides can perform many of the duties previously reserved for doctors.

However, about 60% of people in need of treatment today are not receiving it. The number of people in need of treatment will significantly increase with the expected revision of WHO [World Health Organization] guidelines which may recommend, in line with current evidence, that treatment be initiated earlier in a patient's disease progression. Starting treatment earlier will greatly reduce the risk of tuberculosis infections, among others.

The Need for Political Will

Extending ARV treatment in developing countries to all people in need, while ensuring patients can survive with HIV in the long term, will require much more investment and political will. For treatment to be most successful, patients need to be monitored effectively and have access to newer and more potent drugs when they inevitably develop resistance or side effects to their medicines over time. But most newer drugs are unaffordable because they are protected by patents and crucial monitoring tests are not adapted for use in resource-poor settings.

Over the last decade, effective action by public interest groups and People Living with HIV/AIDS (PLHA) networks has raised the alarm and billions of dollars have been mobilised. However, the international AIDS effort is at a critical juncture, compromised further by the response of world leaders to the economic crisis: The two main funding sources for HIV/AIDS in developing countries, the Global Fund and the U.S.

> **FAST FACT**
>
> An untreated HIV-infected person will progress to AIDS within ten years of becoming infected, according to the Joint United Nations Programme on HIV/AIDS.

President's Emergency Plan for AIDS Relief (PEPFAR), will not be able to support the treatment scale-up at its current rate given insufficient donor commitment. The Global Fund is facing a significant financing gap and PEPFAR's funding levels are flat.

Given the unprecedented disease burden represented by HIV and the proportion of overall mortality caused by AIDS in most affected countries—including child and maternal deaths—HIV/AIDS continues to be a global emergency. An effective HIV/AIDS response, in particular access to treatment, has a positive population-level impact on adult, infant and under-five mortality.

Ensuring Swifter Access to Medicines

Only three years after world leaders met at the 2006 United Nations General Assembly and committed to universal access to HIV prevention, treatment and care, political and funding support is waning.

The number of people who will need treatment by 2030 has been projected to reach as many as 55 million. A sustained response to HIV/AIDS includes an obligation to put people on treatment and to continue treatment as medically required.

To ensure that funds stretch as far as possible to meet the needs, policy actions are needed to contain the cost of drugs, while ensuring quality treatment for the long term.

One of the most promising developments over the past year has been the work of the international drug purchase facility UNITAID to establish a patent pool for AIDS medicines. This would help overcome patent barriers and ensure swifter access to needed medicines at affordable prices, while boosting innovation for new fixed-dose combinations and paediatric formulations. All effort must now be undertaken to ensure the pharmaceutical industry participates and makes this groundbreaking mechanism the lifesaver it is intended to be. . . .

No Time to Scale Back

It is critical that HIV/AIDS continues to be treated as the emergency it is. Funding levels must be increased to take on the massive task of providing sustained AIDS treatment in developing countries. The worrying trend of treatment providers needing to scale back ART at a time when they should be scaling up must be countered with sustained and reaffirmed commitment by leaders and donors to universal access to HIV/AIDS treatment.

EVALUATING THE AUTHOR'S ARGUMENTS:

Doctors Without Borders is a humanitarian organization well known for its work in providing international medical aid. How does your awareness of this group's credentials affect your appraisal of this viewpoint?

Viewpoint

6

Gender Inequality Must Be Challenged

Barbara Crossette

In the following viewpoint Barbara Crossette maintains that the UN has not supported female sexual and reproductive health and rights as it should and that women's health worldwide has suffered as a result of that persisting disempowerment—as can be seen in the death tolls of women from AIDS. Crossette supports the establishment of a UN women's agency and the efforts of Margaret Chan, director-general of the World Health Organization, to make women's health a priority. Crossette also suggests that the vastly different health needs of women in rich countries may make it difficult for the UN to understand and address the health needs of women in poor countries. A former foreign correspondent for *The New York Times,* Barbara Crossette is the author of several books on Asia, including *The Great Hill Stations of Asia.*

"[T]he World Health Organization said . . . that the leading cause of death for girls and women aged fifteen to forty-four is now AIDS."

1. According to Crossette, how long had the United Nations been putting off the establishment of a new woman's agency, at the time of writing?
2. What is "mainstreaming" and how was it implemented with regard to women's health and rights, according to Crossette?
3. What is UNICEF and why has it been an active supporter of women's health?

In a global health report that speaks as much to the powerlessness of women as it does to the diseases that are killing them, the World Health Organization [WHO] said this week [November 10, 2009] that the leading cause of death for girls and women aged 15 to 44 is now AIDS. The report also found that in poor countries, unsafe sex and lack of contraception is the single leading risk factor for death and disability, resulting in unsafe abortion and a range of infections including HIV. Domestic violence poses an additional risk to sexual and reproductive health.

Studies like the WHO report highlight the critical intersections between women's disempowerment and health outcomes—issues the United Nations desperately needs to focus on. But for more than five years, the UN has been dancing around a proposal to create a high-powered, well-financed agency for the world's women. In a last-minute decision in September, before the start of a new UN year, the final session of last year's General Assembly approved the step in principle. But nothing concrete has happened since, and there are plenty of UN members willing to stall implementation, at least into next year.

Progressives may well ask, Didn't the idea of ghettoizing women's issues go out with newspapers' women's pages? That was also the theory around the United Nations, where for decades the buzzword was "mainstreaming," meaning that women would be factored into all the work of the organization. As it turned out, a majority of nations among the UN's 192 members never took seriously the concept of mainstreaming female sexual and reproductive health and rights in development, though the status of women is widely acknowledged to be critical to progress on many fronts from the economy to the environment.

No mention of reproductive rights, aside from maternal health, appears in the Millennium Development Goals, the eight-point plan for reducing poverty and disease worldwide. Ever since the 1994 UN Conference on Population and Development in Cairo, a relentless Vatican campaign aligned with a claque of nations—among them some in which women most need good reproductive healthcare and rights of all kinds—continues to scaremonger. In its sloganeering, gender equality and sexual/reproductive rights become code words for abortion, feminism and lesbianism.

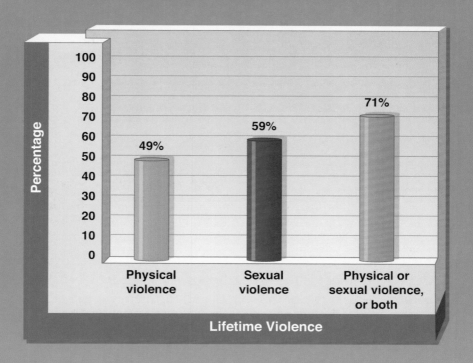

Percentage of Women Who Experienced Violence by an Intimate Partner, Among Ever-Partnered Women Aged 15 to 49 in Butajira, Ethiopia

Lifetime Violence

Taken from: World Health Organization, "WHO Multi-country Study on Women's Health and Domestic Violence Against Women," www.who.int/en.

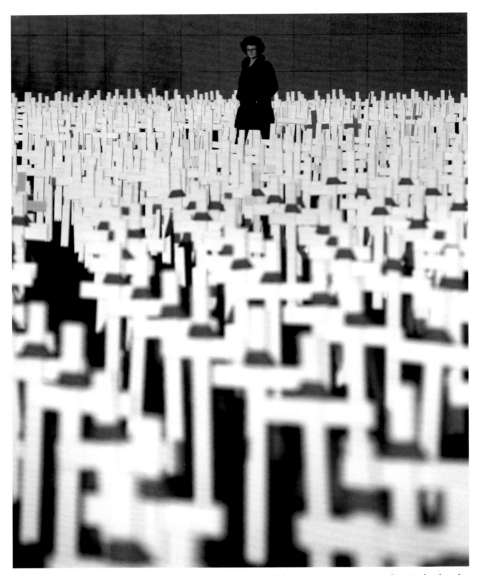

A woman stands amid five thousand crosses at a World AIDS Day event in the Netherlands. In the world today, HIV/AIDS is the leading cause of death among women aged fifteen to forty-four.

The debate over gender rights exposes deep fissures in the UN system. One of them is the divide between the expert UN agencies, bodies staffed largely by professionals, and the majority-rules General Assembly, which can box in the international civil servants of the Secretariat and constrain even a secretary general. In the weeks before he resigned in 2006, Kofi Annan tried to jump-start the creation of the new women's agency and was slapped down by member governments. (Among the opponents at the time were large and important nations such as the United States and India.)

Annan's successor, Ban Ki-moon, got the message and shied away from action when he took office at the beginning of 2007, turning the issue over to the Assembly, a surefire way to stall something innovative. Does this sound like the American healthcare debate?

On the other side of this UN divide are the autonomous or semi-autonomous UN agencies where policies are set and decisions made with less political pressure. When Margaret Chan, a former director of health in Hong Kong, took over as director-general of WHO in 2007, she vowed that women's health would be a priority, and she has been active on that front. So, to varying degrees, have the leaders of the UN Development Fund for Women (UNIFEM), the Population Fund (UNFPA) and UNICEF, the children's fund.

UNICEF? Yes, because teens and even younger girls barely beyond puberty are dying by the thousands in unwanted pregnancies when their small bodies are not developed enough to give birth. Pregnancy-related complications are a leading cause of death among 15- to 19-year-old girls in the developing world. Globally, girls are also victims of sexual abuse at a rate three times that of boys, WHO found.

When Chan released the new report, *Women and Health: Today's Evidence, Tomorrow's Agenda*, on November 9 [2009], she explained why she commissioned it: "I did so based on my conviction that the health of women has been neglected, that this neglect is a major impediment to development, and that the situation needs to improve. I did so based on my conviction that women matter in ways far beyond their role as mothers."

Another fissure that can impede concerted action in the United Nations on women's health and sexual rights yawns between the

> **FAST FACT**
>
> Sub-Saharan Africa is home to 67 percent of all people living with HIV worldwide, according to the Joint United Nations Programme on HIV/AIDS.

health and rights of women in the industrial countries and the global South. Those in Europe or North America who may be surprised to learn that, numerically, HIV/AIDS kills the most women worldwide may also be those in the developed world who do not see the lack of access to contraception (and thus control over their bodies) that poor women endure.

Where women's health is concerned, there are clearly two worlds. The new WHO report, for example, finds that while unwanted pregnancies and unsafe abortion are major killers of young women in poorer countries, the leading cause of death among girls 10 to 19 in rich countries is traffic accidents.

Among adult women, mostly between the ages of 20 and 59, cervical cancer among the poor account for 80 percent of world cases, and most of the deaths. Ninety-nine percent of the more than half a million maternal deaths annually occur in low-income nations, where societal pressures may also contribute to the powerlessness of women. Leading causes of death among the poor include respiratory infections and diarrheal diseases. For women in rich nations, heart disease, stroke and Alzheimer's or other dementias are at the top of the mortality list.

EVALUATING THE AUTHOR'S ARGUMENTS:

Barbara Crossette believes that the establishment of a United Nations women's agency is one of the best ways for the UN to promote women's sexual and reproductive health and rights. Do you agree? Include evidence from this viewpoint with which you agree or disagree.

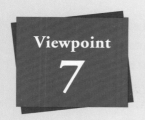
Homophobia Must Be Challenged

amfAR, The Foundation for AIDS Research, International Gay and Lesbian Human Rights Commission, and Human Rights Watch

"To reduce HIV incidence among men who have sex with men, it is essential to confront, condemn, and eradicate . . . homophobia."

The following viewpoint is a declaration of commitment made by amfAR, The Foundation for AIDS Research, the International Gay and Lesbian Human Rights Commission, and Human Rights Watch on the International Day Against Homophobia on May 17, 2008. These authors contend that one of the biggest obstacles to HIV prevention and treatment is discrimination against people on the basis of sexual orientation or identity. Violence and stigma against same-sex sexual behavior often prevents people from seeking or receiving necessary HIV support services, they argue. The organizations signing this document have agreed to advocate for the rights of lesbian, gay, bisexual, and transgender populations and to educate the public about the connection between homophobia and the spread of HIV.

"All human beings are born free and equal in dignity and rights."

This simple, yet powerful, statement is enshrined in Article 1 of the Universal Declaration of Human Rights, promulgated 60 years ago this year [2008] by the General Assembly of the United Nations. Yet the fundamental right of all human beings to equality and dignity is routinely denied to members of lesbian, gay, bisexual, and transgender communities. Of the 192 member states of the United Nations, 85 have laws that criminalize homosexual conduct, which in some instances is punishable by death.

Violence, rape, harassment, abuse, beating, and even murder, on the basis of sexual orientation or identity, occur around the world with shocking regularity and impunity. Family and friends often ostracize and cast out people, including women and children, who do not conform to social and cultural norms of gender or sexuality, leading to devastating economic disempowerment as well as isolation. Members of lesbian, gay, bisexual and transgender populations are often arrested without cause, imprisoned, and subjected to sexual abuse and/or mandatory HIV testing and anal or vaginal examinations. Discrimination is frequently institutionalized or state sanctioned, whereby law enforcement officials perpetrate human rights violations with impunity or react with indifference to violence based on sexual orientation or gender identity. Attempts to overcome such discrimination, such as gay pride activities or advocacy are opposed or prohibited.

The Impact of Stigma

The negative impact that homophobia has on effective responses to HIV and other sexually transmitted infections is well established.

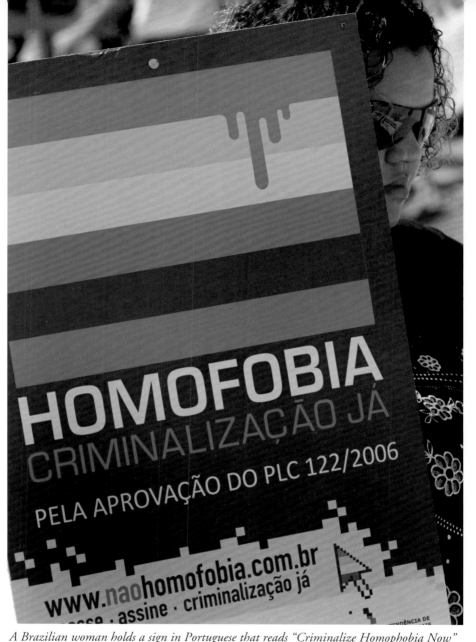

A Brazilian woman holds a sign in Portuguese that reads "Criminalize Homophobia Now" during the first National March Against Homophobia in May 2010.

Even in countries without legal prohibitions against same-sex sexual behavior, widespread stigma often prevents men who have sex with men from seeking or receiving essential HIV prevention, treatment, care and support services. In many cases—particularly in countries where political or social leaders deny the existence of same sex sexuality or criminalize it—these services are absent altogether. Women who deploy their sexualities in ways outside heterosexual social norms may face double burdens of stigma and invisibility. In addition, insufficient research has been conducted on the health care needs of lesbian and bisexual women. Without information, education, support or access to health services, many people unknowingly engage in behaviors, or are placed in situations, that increase their risk of HIV infection and/or unwittingly pass on the virus.

As a result, HIV infection rates remain disproportionately high among men who have sex with men in both developed and developing countries. To reduce HIV incidence among men who have sex with men, it is essential to confront, condemn, and eradicate the homophobia that is the single biggest obstacle to effective HIV prevention, treatment, and care.

A Declaration

It was over eighteen years ago that the World Health Organization removed homosexuality from its list of diseases [in 1990]. The anniversary of that belated act, May 17, is now commemorated as the International Day Against Homophobia. On this day, we, the undersigned, declare zero tolerance for homophobia. We condemn the deafening silence with which nations greet the violence, persecution, discrimination and denial that are perpetrated on lesbian, gay, bisexual and transgender people—a silence that condones the continued violation of the fundamental human rights of these people.

We therefore commit ourselves to the following actions:

1. *Stand up for the human rights and dignity of lesbian, gay, bisexual and transgender (LGBT) populations.*

We commit to undertake, incorporate, and expand the following actions and activities:

1.1 Call for the end of impunity [freedom from punishment] for those who violate the rights of members of LGBT populations;

1.2 Educate and share information with LGBT communities about their human rights and about effective methods of documenting and advocating against violations of their rights;

1.3 Promote the human rights of all people affected by HIV/AIDS in collaboration with LGBT organizations and other human rights organizations;

1.4 Promote access to justice for individuals whose rights have been violated, including access to legal assistance;

1.5 Educate Parliamentarians, the Judiciary, and Ministries of Justice personnel, including police, about their obligations to respect and protect the human rights of all citizens;

1.6 Promote the dissemination and application of the International Guidelines on HIV/AIDS and Human Rights and the Yogyakarta Principles, a document that affirms binding international legal standards for the protection of human rights in relation to sexual orientation and gender identity.

2. *Speak out against homophobia and advocate equal rights for LGBT populations.*

We commit to undertake, incorporate, and/or expand the following actions and activities:

2.1 Advocate policies and programs to fight homophobia at all levels of society, including in the workplace, in educational and healthcare systems, sports and recreation, correctional facilities, and the military and uniformed services;

2.2 Communicate with mass media about the pervasive effects of homophobia, its link to the spread of HIV infection, and the need to fight it at all levels.

2.3 Find and support champions against homophobia and collect examples of successful campaigns against homophobia.

3. *Continue to assert the connection between human rights violations and the spread of HIV infection and other sexually transmitted diseases.*

We commit to undertake, incorporate, and/or expand the following actions and activities:

Countries with Laws Banning Homosexual Activity

Country				
Afghanistan	Algeria	Angola	Bahrain	Bangladesh
Barbados	Benin	Bhutan	Botswana	Brunei
Burma (Myanmar)	Burundi	Cameroon	Cape Verde	Cook Islands
Djibouti	Ethiopia	Fiji	French Polynesia (Tahiti)	Ghana
Grenada	Guinea	Guyana	India	Iran*
Jamaica	Kenya	Kiribati	Kuwait	Laos
Lebanon	Liberia	Libya	Malawi	Maldives Islands
Malaysia	Mali	Marshall Islands	Mauritania*	Mauritius
Mongolia	Morocco	Mozambique	Namibia	Nauru
Nepal	Nicaragua	Nigeria*	Niue	Oman
Pakistan*	Papua New Guinea	Puerto Rico	Qatar	Saint Lucia
Samoa	Saudi Arabia*	Senegal	Seychelles Islands	Sierra Leone
Singapore	Solomon Islands	Somalia	Sri Lanka	Sudan*
Swaziland	Syria	Tajikstan	Tanzania	Tokelau
Togo	Tonga	Trinidad and Tobago	Tunisia	Tuvalu
Uganda	United Arab Emirates	Uzbekistan	Yemen*	Zambia
Zimbabwe				

*Countries where homosexual acts are punishable by death

Taken from: "Homosexual Rights Around the World," www.asylumlaw.org, October 12, 2006.

3.1 Promote the dissemination and application of relevant provisions of the International Guidelines on HIV/AIDS;

3.2 Promote continuing research into effective programs that link human rights protection and empowerment with effective community responses to HIV;

3.3 Promote the continuing development of means by which to measure and monitor these populations and their health and human rights needs.

EVALUATING THE AUTHORS' ARGUMENTS:

The authors of this selection maintain that promoting the human rights and dignity of lesbian, gay, bisexual, and transgender people will help to curtail the global AIDS epidemic. Do you agree with their views? Why or why not? Use supporting evidence from the viewpoints in this text in defending your answer.

Facts About AIDS

Editor's note: These facts can be used in reports or papers to reinforce or add credibility when making important points or claims.

Basic Facts About HIV/AIDS

According to The Foundation for AIDS Research:

- HIV is carried in blood, semen, vaginal secretions, and breast milk.
- HIV is transmitted through:
    - unprotected sexual intercourse, vaginal or anal;
    - unprotected oral sex;
    - sharing needles or syringes with someone who is HIV positive;
    - infection during pregnancy, childbirth, or breast-feeding;
    - contact with HIV infected blood or semen through a cut or sore in the skin.
- HIV is not transmitted through:
    - sharing food or eating utensils,
    - the air by coughing or sneezing,
    - hugging and kissing,
    - sweat,
    - sharing bathroom facilities,
    - insect bites,
    - donating blood for a blood bank.
- HIV risk is reduced by
    - the use of latex condoms during every sexual act,
    - abstinence.

AIDS in the United States

According to the Centers for Disease Control and Prevention:

- More than 1 million Americans are living with AIDS.
- One out of five HIV-positive Americans are unaware of their infection.
- About fifty-six thousand Americans become newly infected with HIV each year.

- More than eighteen thousand people die of AIDS each year in the United States.
- Those infected through heterosexual contact account for 31 percent of annual new infections and 28 percent of those living with HIV.
- Women account for 27 percent of annual new HIV infections and 25 percent of those living with HIV.
- Intravenous drug users account for 12 percent of new HIV infections and 19 percent of those living with HIV.
- Men who have sex with men account for 53 percent of annual new HIV infections and 48 percent of people living with HIV.

The Global AIDS Epidemic

According to Joint United Nations Programme on HIV/AIDS:
- 33.4 million people are living with HIV/AIDS.
- The number of women living with HIV/AIDS is 15.7 million.
- The number of children under age fifteen living with HIV/AIDS is 2.1 million.
- 2.7 million adults were newly infected with HIV in 2008.
- In 2008, 430,000 children under age fifteen were newly infected with HIV.
- In 2008, 2 million adults died of AIDS.
- In 2008, 280,000 children under age fifteen died of AIDS.
- More than 8,000 people die of AIDS daily.
- Since the beginning of the epidemic, 60 million people have contracted HIV and at least 25 million have died of AIDS-related causes.
- Sixty-seven percent of all people living with HIV (22 million) live in sub-Saharan Africa.
- Ninety-one percent of the world's HIV-positive children live in sub-Saharan Africa.
- Asia and the Pacific have 4 million people living with HIV/AIDS.
- The Caribbean has 240,000 people living with HIV/AIDS.
- Latin America has 2 million people living with HIV/AIDS.
- North Africa and the Middle East have 310,000 people living with HIV/AIDS.
- Eastern Europe and Central Asia have 1.5 million people living with HIV/AIDS.
- Western and Central Europe have 850,000 people living with HIV/AIDS.

According to AVERT:

- In developing countries 9.5 million people are in immediate need of lifesaving AIDS drugs; of these, 4 million (42 percent) are receiving the drugs.
- Africa has over 14 million AIDS orphans.
- Eleven percent of worldwide HIV infections are among babies who acquire the virus from their mothers.
- Ten percent of worldwide HIV infections are caused by intravenous drug use.
- Five to 10 percent of worldwide HIV infections are due to men having sex with men.
- Five to 10 percent of worldwide HIV infections occur in health-care settings.
- Globally, two-thirds of new infections occur through heterosexual intercourse.
- AIDS is the second-most common cause of death for twenty- to twenty-four-year-olds.

Organizations to Contact

The editors have compiled the following list of organizations concerned with the issues debated in this book. The descriptions are derived from materials provided by the organizations. All have publications or information available for interested readers. The list was compiled on the date of publication of the present volume; the information provided here may change. Be aware that many organizations take several weeks or longer to respond to inquiries, so allow as much time as possible for the receipt of requested materials.

AIDS Vaccine Advocacy Coalition (AVAC)
101 W. Twenty-third St., #2227, New York, NY 10011
(212) 367-1279
fax: (646) 365-3452
e-mail: avac@avac.org
website: www.avac.org

AVAC is a community- and consumer-based organization founded in 1995 to accelerate the ethical development and global delivery of vaccines for HIV/AIDS. The organization provides independent analysis, policy advocacy, public education, and mobilization to enhance AIDS research. It also provides the quarterly update *PxWire* and *The AIDS Vaccine Handbook*.

Alive and Well AIDS Alternatives
11684 Ventura Blvd., Studio City, CA 91604
(818) 780-1875
fax: (818) 780-7093
e-mail: info@aliveandwell.org
website: www.aliveandwell.org

Alive and Well AIDS Alternatives challenges popular beliefs and theories about HIV and AIDS. It sponsors clinical studies and scientific research in an attempt to verify the central tenets about the disease, its cause, and its treatments. The organization publishes the book *What If Everything You Thought You Knew About AIDS Was Wrong?*

American Red Cross AIDS Education Office
1730 D St. NW, Washington, DC 20006
(202) 737-8300
website: www.redcross.org

Established in 1881, the American Red Cross is one of America's oldest public health organizations. Its AIDS Education Office publishes pamphlets, brochures, and posters containing facts about AIDS. These materials are available at local Red Cross chapters. In addition, many chapters offer informational videotapes, conduct presentations, and operate speakers' bureaus.

Center for Women Policy Studies (CWPS)
1776 Massachusetts Ave. NW, Ste. 450, Washington, DC 20036
(202) 872-1770
fax: (202) 296-8962
e-mail: cwps@centerwomenpolicy.org
website: www.centerwomenpolicy.org

The CWPS was the first national policy institute to focus specifically on issues affecting the social, legal, and economic status of women. It believes that the government and the medical community have neglected the effect of AIDS on women and that more action should be taken to help women who are infected with HIV. Its website includes the National Resource Center on Women and AIDS Policy, an archive of links to publications such as "Inaccessible Miracles? Women's Access to HIV/AIDS Medications."

Centers for Disease Control and Prevention (CDC)
National Prevention Information Network (NPIN)
PO Box 6003, Rockville, MD 20849-6003
(800) 458-5231
fax: (888) 282-7681
e-mail: info@cdcnpin.org
website: www.cdcnpin.org

The CDC is the US government agency charged with protecting the public health by preventing and controlling diseases and by responding to public health emergencies. The CDC National Prevention Information Network is a reference and referral service for information on HIV/AIDS, viral hepatitis, sexually transmitted diseases, and tuberculosis. The NPIN's services are designed to facilitate the sharing of information and resources among people working locally and internationally for the prevention and treatment of these diseases. Its website offers links to articles, reports, and social marketing campaigns, including *Prevention Is Care.*

Family Research Council (FRC)
801 G St. NW, Washington, DC 20001
(800) 225-4008 • (202) 393-2100
fax: (202) 393-2134
website: www.frc.org

The FRC promotes the traditional family unit and conventional Judeo-Christian values. The council opposes the public education system's tolerance of homosexuality and condom distribution programs, which its members believe encourage sexual promiscuity and lead to the spread of AIDS. It publishes numerous reports, pamphlets, and articles from a conservative perspective, including "Spending Too Little on Abstinence" and "Why Wait: The Benefits of Abstinence Until Marriage."

The Foundation for AIDS Research (amfAR)
120 Wall St., 13th Fl., New York, NY 10005-3908
(212) 806-1600
fax: (212) 806-1601
website: www.amfar.org

In 1985 the American Foundation for AIDS Research was formed through the unification of the AIDS Medical Foundation and the National AIDS Research Foundation. In 2005 amfAR became simply The Foundation for AIDS Research. The organization supports AIDS prevention and research and advocates AIDS-related public policy. It publishes several monographs, compendiums, journals, and periodicals, including the semiannual newsletter *Innovations* and the handbook *Are You Positive You're Negative?*

Global AIDS Interfaith Alliance (GAIA)
The Presidio of San Francisco, PO Box 29110, San Francisco, CA 94129-0110

(415) 461-7196
fax: (415) 461-9681
e-mail: info@thegaia.org
website: www.thegaia.org

GAIA is a nonprofit organization composed of AIDS researchers and doctors, religious leaders, and African medical officials, most of whom are associated with religiously based clinics and hospitals. The organization is concerned with infrastructure development and the training of prevention educators and personnel to conduct HIV testing and counseling. It also emphasizes the modification of values, structures, and practices that predispose women and girls to higher HIV infection rates than men, that stigmatize ill persons, and that contribute to public denial. GAIA's website offers news and updates about AIDS.

International AIDS Vaccine Initiative (IAVI)

110 William St., 27th Fl., New York, NY 10038
(212) 847-1111
website: www.iavi.org

IAVI is a global organization working to speed the development and distribution of preventative AIDS vaccines. IAVI's work focuses on mobilizing support through advocacy and education, acceleration of scientific progress, encouraging industrial participation in AIDS vaccine development, and assuring global access to the vaccines once they are developed. IAVI publishes policy papers and articles such as "Spotlight: A Boost for African Science." Its website includes a news center with links to fact sheets, press releases, and media resources.

International Council of AIDS Service Organizations (ICASO)

65 Wellesley St. East, Ste. 403, Toronto, ON M4Y 1G7 Canada
(416) 921-0018
fax: (416) 921-9979
e-mail: icaso@icaso.org
website: www.icaso.org

ICASO's mission is to mobilize and support diverse community organizations to build an effective global response to HIV and AIDS. It recognizes human rights as being central to an intelligent public health strategy to combat the epidemic. Operating globally, regionally, and locally, ICASO gathers and disseminates information on key issues and advocates for universal access to comprehensive HIV/AIDS services. Its website provides links to policy papers and community research reports, including "Voice and Visibility: Frontline Perspectives on How the Global News Media Reports on HIV/AIDS."

Joint United Nations Programme on HIV/AIDS (UNAIDS)
20 Ave. Appia, CH-1211, Geneva 27, Switzerland
(4122) 791-3666
fax: (4122) 791-4187
website: www.unaids.org

UNAIDS is a joint United Nations program on HIV/AIDS created by the combination of six organizations. It is a leading advocate for world-wide action against HIV/AIDS. Its global mission is to lead, strengthen, and support an expanded response to the AIDS epidemic that will prevent the spread of HIV, provide care and support for those infected and affected by HIV/AIDS, and alleviate the socioeconomic and human impact of the epidemic. UNAIDS has many publications available on its website, including *Monitoring the Declaration of Commitment on HIV/AIDS* and *Crisis, Opportunity, and Transformation: AIDS Response at a Crossroads.*

National AIDS Fund (NAF)
1424 K St. NW, 2nd Fl., Washington, DC 20005
(202) 408-4848
fax: (202) 408-1818
e-mail: info@aidsfund.org
website: www.aidsfund.org

The NAF seeks to eliminate HIV as a major health and social problem. Its members work in partnership with the public and private sectors to provide care and to prevent new infections in communities and in the workplace by means of advocacy, grants, research, and education. The fund publishes the *NAF Quarterly Newsletter* and provides links to press releases, fact sheets, and testing resources.

National Association of People with AIDS (NAPWA)
8401 Colesville Rd., Ste. 505, Silver Spring, MD 20910
(240) 247-0880 • (866) 846-7366

fax: (240) 247-0574

e-mail: development@napwa.org

website: www.napwa.org

The NAPWA is a nonprofit organization that represents people with HIV. Its members believe that it is the inalienable right of every person with HIV to have health care, be free from discrimination, have the right to a dignified death, be adequately housed, be protected from violence, and travel and immigrate regardless of country of origin or HIV status. The association publishes the bimonthly newsletter *Positive Voice* and offers links to HIV-testing promotional materials and an annual report.

For Further Reading

Books

Engel, Jonathan. *The Epidemic: A Global History of AIDS.* Washington, DC: Smithsonian, 2006. Engel presents an overview of the history, spread, and consequences of HIV, examining the virus as a worldwide phenomenon.

Epstein, Helen. *The Invisible Cure: Why We Are Losing the Fight Against AIDS in Africa.* New York: Picador, 2008. A public health specialist and molecular biologist argues that inefficient medical bureaucracies and social structures have contributed to the spread of AIDS in Africa. In Epstein's opinion, Africans often have better ideas about addressing AIDS in their own communities than Western philanthropists do.

Holleran, Andrew. *Chronicle of a Plague, Revisited: AIDS and Its Aftermath.* New York: Da Capo, 2008. A series of twenty-four essays that explores the devastating impact of the AIDS epidemic on the US gay community and in the larger global arena as well.

Hunter, Susan. *AIDS in America.* New York: Palgrave Macmillan, 2009. A consultant to UNICEF maintains that AIDS is becoming more common and potentially more deadly.

Lyon, Maureen E., and Lawrence J. D'Angelo, eds. *Teenagers, HIV and AIDS: Insights from Youths Living with the Virus.* Santa Barbara, CA: ABC-CLIO, 2006. This book combines information on the biology, prevention, and treatment of HIV infection with the experiences of youths who tell readers what it is like to live with HIV/AIDS.

Mugyenyi, Peter. *Genocide by Denial: How Profiteering from HIV/AIDS Killed Millions.* Kamapala, Uganda: Fountain, 2008. This author charges that the wealth-seeking pharmaceutical companies of the West responded far too slowly to the global AIDS crisis. He calls for rapid access to lifesaving drugs and ethical treatment of the HIV-infected poor.

Nolen, Stephanie. *28 Stories of AIDS in Africa.* New York: Walker, 2008. The author offers twenty-eight portraits of Africans affected by HIV, putting a human face on the AIDS epidemic in Africa.

Steinberg, Jonny. *Sizwe's Test: A Young Man's Journey Through Africa's AIDS Epidemic.* New York: Simon and Schuster, 2010. A South African journalist seeks to understand why so many people in his native country resist HIV testing and treatment.

Whiteside, Alan. *HIV/AIDS: A Very Short Introduction.* New York: Oxford University Press, 2008. Packed with statistics and scientific explanations, this book investigates the social, political, and economic aspects of HIV, assessing the prevalence and spread of AIDS around the world.

Periodicals and Internet Sources

Barnes, Pamela, and Nicholas Hellman. "This Pandemic Is Entirely Preventable," *Globe and Mail* (Toronto), February 9, 2009.

Bates, Betsy. "Expert Warns of Ominous Signs in AIDS Fight," *Internal Medicine News,* April 1, 2007.

The Body: The Complete HIV/AIDS Resource. "Fact Sheet: Myth Versus Reality," November 2009. www.thebody.com.

Byrnes, Sholto. "Faith, Hope, and Clarity," *New Statesman,* January 2010.

Catholic Insight. "Pope Benedict and the Condom Hysteria," interview with Pope Benedict XVI, May 2009.

Centers for Disease Control and Prevention. "HIV Prevention in the United States at a Critical Crossroads," August 2009. www.cdc.gov.

Economist. "Sex and Sensibility: The Pope in Africa," March 21, 2009.

Freston, Tom. "Media and the HIV Fight," *Adweek,* December 7, 2009.

Gorna, Robin. "Is Universal Access for HIV a Realistic Goal?" *Global Health,* Spring 2010.

Hanson, Carolyn. "A Matter of Life and Death: Homophobia Threatens HIV/AIDS Work in Africa," The Foundation for AIDS Research, April 12, 2010. www.amfar.org.

Human Rights Watch. "A Question of Life or Death," December 16, 2008. www.hrw.org.

Knight, Robert. "AIDS: The Questions They Won't Ask," Townhall, November 30, 2007. http://townhall.com.

Leake, Matthew. "Universal Access to AIDS Treatment: Targets and Challenges," AVERT, June 2009. www.avert.org.

Lubbock-Avalanche Journal (Texas). "Poverty-Stricken Haiti Providing Example for Others in AIDS Fight," July 17, 2009.

Meldrum, Andrew. "AIDS Activist Turns South Africa Around," *Progressive*, May 2007.

Muga, Wycliffe. "When Public Negligence Can Become Criminal," *African Business*, May 2009.

New York Times. "The Global AIDS Fight," February 29, 2008.

Piot, Peter. "Combatting AIDS: What More Needs to Be Done?" *UN Chronicle*, December 2007.

Pisani, Elizabeth. "This Is the Worst Kind of Good News," *The Times* (London), September 25, 2009.

Roberts, Deborah. "My Firsthand View of AIDS in Africa," *Ebony*, January 2007.

Seymour, Richard. "Step Out of the Dark Ages," *Middle East*, July 2008.

Sidibe, Michel. "This Is Our Zero Hour," UNAIDS, July 18, 2010. www.unaids.org.

Weinstein, Steve. "The Next Condom Conundrum: Why Use a Rubber When You Can Just Pop a Pill?" *Advocate*, February 2009.

World Health Organization, UNICEF, and UNAIDS. *Towards Universal Access: Scaling Up Priority HIV/AIDS Interventions in the Health Sector*, September 2010. www.who.int/hiv/en.

York, Geoffrey. "G8's Maternal Health Initiative Neglects AIDS Funding," *Globe and Mail* (Toronto), May 28, 2010.

Index

Picture Credits

AP Images/Frank Franklin II, 75

AP Images/Sakchai Lalit, 64

AP Images/George Osodi, 77

AP Images/Eraldo Peres, 111

AP Images/Khalil Senosi, 95

AP Images/Waldo Swiegers, 91

AP Images/Schalk van Zuydam, 68

BSIP/Photo Researchers, Inc., 71

Marco Di Lauro/Getty Images, 54

Jeff Fusco/Getty Images, 41

Romeo Gacad/AFP/Getty Images, 33

Gale/Cengage Learning, 14, 19, 35, 39, 44, 48, 53, 60, 65, 73, 79, 84, 96, 105, 113 Wairimu Gitani/Reuters/Landov, 100

Uletl Ifansasti/Getty Images, 43

Matt Jones/The Washington Times/Landov, 59

Jerry Lampen/Reuters/Landov, 106

© Jake Lyell/Alamy, 29

Frank May/dpa/Landov, 83

John Mottern/AFP/Getty Images, 17

© PHOTOTAKE, Inc./Alamy, 10

Chris Sattlberger/Photo Researchers, Inc., 23

Sergei Supinsky/AFP/Getty Images, 13